# WOMEN AND MEN

## *New Perspectives on Gender Differences*

ISSUES IN
PSYCHIATRY

*Joseph D. Bloom, M.D.*
*Series Editor*

# WOMEN AND MEN

## New Perspectives on Gender Differences

Edited by

*Malkah T. Notman, M.D.*
Clinical Professor of Psychiatry
Harvard Medical School
Director of Academic Affairs
The Cambridge Hospital
Cambridge, Massachusetts

*Carol C. Nadelson, M.D.*
Professor and Vice Chair of Academic Affairs
Department of Psychiatry
Tufts University School of Medicine
Director of Training and Education
Department of Psychiatry
New England Medical Center Hospitals
Boston, Massachusetts

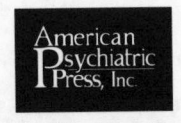

American
Psychiatric
Press, Inc.

Washington, DC
London, England

Note: Books published by the American Psychiatric Press, Inc., represent the views and opinions of the individual authors and do not necessarily represent the policies and opinions of the Press or the American Psychiatric Association.

American Psychiatric Press, Inc.
1400 K Street, N.W., Washington, DC  20005

The paper used in this publication meets the minimum requirements of the American National Standard for Information Sciences—Permanence of Paper for Printed Library Materials, ANSI Z39.48-1984.                    ∞

**Library of Congress Cataloging-in-Publication Data**

Women and men: new perspectives on gender differences / edited by Malkah
   T. Notman, Carol C. Nadelson. — 1st ed.
      p.      cm. — (Issues in psychiatry)
      Includes bibliographical references.
      ISBN 0-88048-136-6 (alk. paper)
      1. Sex differences (Psychology)  2. Sex role.  I. Notman, Malkah
   T.  II. Nadelson, Carol C.  III. Series.
      [DNLM: 1. Identification (Psychology)  2. Men.  3. Sex Characteris-
   tics.  4. Women.      HQ1075 W872]
   BF692.2.W65      1990
   155.3'3—dc20
   DNLM/DLC
   for Library of Congress                                            90-548
                                                                        CIP


**British Library Cataloguing in Publication Data**

A CIP record is available from the British Library.

# Contents

# Contributors

**Jessie Bernard, Ph.D.**
Research Scholar, Honoris Causa
Pennsylvania State University
State College, Pennsylvania

**Ruth Bleier, Ph.D.**
Professor of Neurophysiology
Professor of Women's Studies Program
University of Wisconsin
Madison, Wisconsin

**Virginia L. Clower, M.D.**
Psychoanalyst
Clinical Professor of Psychiatry
Medical College of Virginia
Richmond, Virginia

**Carol Gilligan, Ph.D.**
Professor of Education
Harvard Graduate School of Education
Harvard University
Cambridge, Massachusetts

**Hilda Kahne, Ph.D.**
Professor of Economics
Wheaton College
Norton, Massachusetts

**Robert A. LeVine, Ph.D.**
Roy E. Larsen Professor of Education and Human Development
Department of Anthropology
Harvard University
Cambridge, Massachusetts

**Bruce S. McEwen, Ph.D.**
Professor and Head of Laboratory of Endocrinology
Rockefeller University
New York, New York

**Carol C. Nadelson, M.D.**
Professor and Vice Chair of Academic Affairs
Department of Psychiatry
Tufts University School of Medicine
Director of Training and Education
Department of Psychiatry
New England Medical Center Hospitals
Boston, Massachusetts

**Malkah T. Notman, M.D.**
Clinical Professor of Psychiatry
Harvard Medical School
Director of Academic Affairs
The Cambridge Hospital
Cambridge, Massachusetts

**Nancy Felipe Russo, Ph.D.**
Director of Women's Studies
Professor of Psychology
Arizona State University
Tempe, Arizona

# Introduction

In the past two decades, research findings from the biological sciences, the social sciences, and psychology have contributed to the evolution of new ideas and concepts. The expansion of knowledge in the neurosciences has changed our understanding of how the brain functions and to some extent how brain and mind are related. One important area of increased investigation concerns gender differences.

Many societal realities have changed during the past two decades, including the entrance of women into the work force and the increase in variations in family patterns. Reflecting these shifts, many of the problems that women present to clinicians are also different. A number of the theories and constructs that we relied on in the past have been challenged. Our thinking has begun to reflect new research that has raised questions about earlier views, which were themselves stereotypes. New concepts of normality and psychopathology have emerged. Therapeutic goals have changed as norms have shifted. For example, the concept of a woman as "normal" only if she is married and a mother has given way to the recognition of a range of "normal" life-styles.

Many clinicians have not had access to the research findings and have not been exposed to controversies that can shape their clinical judgments. The literature in a number of related fields is often not readily available, and clinicians may not have the background information to accurately assess the differences of opinion reflected in the available data. In this book, we will present perspectives and data from the biological and social sciences that describe the state of research findings and contribute to our current understanding of gender differences, their range and extent, and how they are influenced or even created by social, cultural, and biological factors.

The controversy regarding which gender differences are biologically based and to what extent they determine behavior occurs on many levels. A number of questions occur in thinking about men's and women's roles and their determinants. What are the limits of human adaptation in different societies? What have been the roles of women in societies with varying social organizations? What appear to be the universals? How are gender roles derived? How do these roles relate to physical characteristics, such as an individual's size and strength? How are these roles related to patterns of social organization? How might roles change in the face of new technology and life conditions? What previous adaptations, such as those based on physical strength, have become less salient? To what extent do gender roles reflect underlying biologically determined aptitudes and limitations? These questions arise in many discussions about women, gender roles, the effects of social change, the potential for adaptation, and the etiology of psychopathology. Although these questions obviously cannot be fully answered, these chapters consider many of the pertinent areas that have potential clinical applicability.

In Chapter 1, Dr. Robert LeVine presents an overview of anthropological studies of social roles and family patterns, addressing some of the questions we have raised. He summarizes cross-cultural comparisons of women's and men's roles in a number of societies and reviews the activities that societies have permitted and assigned to women and to men. He presents his views regarding current possibilities of roles and those that might develop in the future.

In Chapter 2, Dr. Hilda Kahne examines the relationship between women's concerns and economic realities and policies. She reviews economic research as it applies to women and correlates work, both inside and outside the home, with life conditions. For example, she considers ongoing income level differences between women and men and relates these variables to family life.

In Chapter 3, we summarize some of the recent research on gender differences in brain structure and function in the neurology and psychology literature.

Some researchers report gender differences in cognitive abilities and in brain anatomy and connect them to observations of personality characteristics and behaviors; others question the validity and generalizability of findings. These differences are often considered biologically determined and are associated with differences in the way women and men are perceived and treated. Assumptions that women and men have vastly different abilities are often stated without regard for the limits of our knowledge and its applicability. Drs. Nancy Russo and Ruth Bleier, in Chapters 5 and 6, respectively, point to a long history in which women's inferior status has been justified on the basis of anatomic brain differences. They caution against allowing the historical tendency to influence the interpretation of data, especially when it appears to document differences in certain skills and abilities that are then connected with different brain structure.

In one sense, the existence of anatomic and physiologic gender differences is obvious and not a matter of dispute. Men and women also have different life experiences. In Chapter 10, Dr. Carol Gilligan reminds us that these differences are an important reality and that we must begin to understand the meanings and effects of differences. What is at issue is the inherent and inevitable nature of these differences and the values assigned to them. If a woman's brain has been developed to control the hormonal fluctuations that govern menstruation, can we extrapolate and assume that differences in basic abilities and skills account for some of the differences in the social roles of men and women? The extent, the basis, and the manner in which the obvious variations between men and women are related to cognitive and neurological differences clearly constitute an extremely controversial area. What are cited as "objective" data can be and have been influenced by preset ideas and faulty methodology. Research questions can be asked in such a way as to confirm expectations. Indeed, even the language used communicates values and beliefs. If we study "masculine" and "feminine" traits, are we directing our conclusions?

Chapter 4, by Dr. Bruce McEwen, provides some data on hormonal determinants of gender behavior from animal studies. Drs. Russo and Bleier review, in their chapters, the data from neurological studies that form the basis of conclusions as to gender differences and raise questions about how research is assessed, particularly findings in mental health and psychological development areas. The results often appear to be contradictory. One criticism of some of the conclusions rests on the leap some researchers make from data about anatomical structures to conclusions about complex mental functions. Because these relationships have not been completely established, specific findings may erroneously lead to generalizations broader than are warranted. Functions that are measured and reported, such as spatial skills, the quality of listening, and the capacity to rotate the image of an object mentally, are "metafunctions" and are traceable only partially and indirectly to neurological structures. These metafunctions involve the integration of many functions because the brain as a whole functions at a level of integration that is not the same as the sum of specific functional parts.

In addition, many of the data about the neurological basis of different abilities have been derived from pathology, particularly from findings of neurological deficits that are the result of injuries or illness; others are from studies measuring isolated characteristics with questionable generalizability. For example, findings from measures of dichotic listening, in which auditory stimuli are provided to each ear differently, have been generalized to conclusions about differences in the functions of the different sides of the brain. Contradictions in results may also exist because the measured populations are different, as are the variables studied and the states of the subjects at the time of the studies.

In this book we have not specifically addressed pharmacological data regarding sex differences, although this is also an important area (see Russo 1985; Vannicelli and Nash 1984). Information about drug effects has generally been obtained from studies of normal males, and many of the potential differences in women have not been taken into account, for example, different biochemical and physiologic processes, different hormonal patterns, and the effect of reproductive events.

Psychoanalytic formulations about women have also changed in response to the scholarship and research of the past two decades. Chapter 9 by Dr. Malkah Notman and Chapter 7 by Dr. Virginia Clower emphasize the need to reconceptualize theories regarding the separate and distinct psychological development of women. Dr. Clower integrates newer observations of children, attending to gender and developmental differences in early experiences, perceptions, conflicts, skills, and interactions. Using as a framework formulations by Mahler regarding the separation-individuation phases of development, Dr. Clower delineates developmental gender differences and their implications for later symptom formation.

If, as Dr. Clower describes, there are different paths of male and female development, associated with different patterns of relationships and attachments, then these paths have important clinical consequences. We might see, for example, the desire to please regarded differently in a man and in a woman in comparable situations. A young woman job applicant being interviewed by a man in a position of authority assumes that she should try to make a good impression; in the process she is attuned to say and do what she believes is expected from her. Is she "overly" concerned with his good opinion and thus not "independent enough"? The judgment of being overly concerned is determined by one's ideas about independence, assertiveness, challenging authority, and their appropriate expression, as well as other factors. We might also say that this woman was taking a "feminine" position in relation to a man in authority. These judgments about normality of personality, style, and behavior are frequently made without conscious awareness of the determinants.

Dr. Jessie Bernard, in Chapter 8, provides a sociological perspective on marriage. She observes the changing patterns and expectations of marriage through the 1970s and early 1980s, noting the historical context and gender differences in expectations and responses.

The changes in marriage and work that are described by Drs. Bernard and Kahne reflect the changing social reality for most families. To judge a family pattern as deviant because it is different from previous patterns and idealized or stereotyped views is a common fallacy. The clinician, knowing that over 50% of women with young children are in the work force, will view a working mother, her options, her choices, and the effects on her children differently than the clinician who practiced a generation ago. Then, the clinician might have focused on attachment problems in children and blamed them on the absent mother, rather than recognizing the social reality and looking more thoroughly at diverse biopsychosocial factors.

All chapters tap into an enormous and evolving body of information. In this book, it is our intent to provide current data and theory and to inform and enlighten the reader about the ongoing controversies in gender-related topics that will require integration and application by the clinician.

Malkah T. Notman, M.D.
Carol C. Nadelson, M.D.

# References

Russo N (ed): A Women's Mental Health Agenda. Washington, DC, American Psychological Association, 1985

Vannicelli M, Nash L: Effect of sex bias on women's studies on alcoholism. Alcoholism: Clinical and Experimental Research 8:334–336, 1984

# Chapter 1

# Gender Differences: Interpreting Anthropological Data

## Robert A. LeVine, Ph.D.

Studies of women and gender have proliferated in the anthropological literature since 1970, providing new opportunities to consider old problems in the light of more adequate data and to find more sophisticated ways of conceptualizing gender differences as social, cultural, and psychological phenomena. The unprecedented number of research publications reflects the influence of the women's movement. Some of the articles and books are stridently feminist in tone, but most are sober, scholarly works that add empirical knowledge or theoretical insight to our understanding of gender in the human species.

Quinn (1977) provides an excellent review through 1976. In the subsequent decade, the literature continued to expand and has not been comprehensively reviewed for this chapter. Much of it concerns economic, political, and cultural conditions of indirect relevance to the focus of this volume. The comparative analysis by Sanday (1981) includes a great deal of ethnographic information as well as a sophisticated interpretation. Monographs by Abu-Lughod (1986) and S. LeVine (1979) explore the emotional experience of women in the non-Western societies of Egypt and Kenya, respectively.

That a literature inspired directly or indirectly by an ideological movement could be scientifically valuable is indeed remarkable. It is attributable in this case to three facts: 1) there was already a vigorous and long-standing tradition of research on women's roles and gender differences in social and cultural anthropology; 2) many leading anthropologists of the older and younger generations were women who concerned themselves with these topics; and 3) the expansion of the anthropological profession as a whole and of its fieldwork opportunities, particularly after 1960, facilitated the collection of a vast amount of data—much of it in settings previously undocumented—that could shed further light on this subject.

This literature on women and gender differences has its limitations, particularly in its relevance to the concerns of psychiatrists. Reflecting dominant intellectual currents in the field as a whole, it contains more about the public positions of women, their economic conditions and activities, and their representations in cultural symbols and ideologies than about their personal experience, their psychological functioning, and their acquisition of gender-specific orientations in childhood. There has been some attention to the latter topics, however, and studies of the socioeconomic and cultural contexts of women's lives have provided an indispensable background for any psychosocial investigation. In this chapter, I present a brief overview of several topics of psychological and developmental interest, and suggest some needs for further research.[1]

## Overview of Anthropological Studies on Gender Differences

This overview does not represent a consensus on the points summarized. Anthropologists who study gender are divided along the same lines that fragment the field as a whole: universalism versus relativism, materialism versus idealism, inclusion versus exclusion of psychological and biological dimensions in the analysis of social and cultural phenomena, and positivistic versus interpretive methods. To expect a consensus from such a divided scientific community would be excessively hopeful even if we were not considering an issue as political as gender. In my own view, however, the evidence available supports the following statements.

First, some basic facts can serve as starting points. Sexual dimorphism in certain adaptive characteristics is universal in human populations. The unique reproductive capacities of females normally mark their lives by menstruation, pregnancy, parturition, lactation, and menopause. Males are, on the average, larger and have greater physical strength than females in the same population. The burden of evidence also indicates that males are more aggressive, although this is not as well established as the facts of physical morphology and reproductive capacity (Quinn 1977). Recurrent gender differences in child behavior exist across diverse cultures: boys 3–6 years of age exhibit more aggression, particularly rough-and-tumble play, than girls, and girls at that age exhibit more touching behavior (Whiting and Edwards 1973). This suggests that males and females are predisposed to divergent behavioral development.

Second, none of these capacities or apparent predispositions are uniformly translated into adaptive outcomes across human populations because of variations in technology, socioeconomic organization, and cultural values. Female reproduction can be foreclosed by celibacy and foreshortened by contraception. Lactation can be avoided by using wet nurses or infant formula. Menopause can pale into ambiguity as a life course marker in low-fertility populations where women cease childbearing 20 or 30 years before the cessation of menses. The strength of males can diminish in its relevance to occupational roles as machinery becomes available to do the heavy work. The aggressiveness of young males, though valuable for defense in a warrior force or militia, can become socially disruptive if there is no need for local troops. Behavioral differences between boys and girls can be reduced in later childhood when they are raised together and boys perform tasks defined as feminine. Thus the existence of gender-specific capacities does not predict how or to what extent they will be used for purposes of adaptation.

Some non-Western cases documented by anthropologists provide striking support for this point. Among peoples of the East African highlands, for example, where plows and draft animals were absent, the heavy work of cultivation was done largely by women using short-handled hoes. The same women routinely carried 50-pound loads on their heads over considerable distances, in addition to bearing and raising children and managing their homes. No a priori concept of women's physical capacities could have forecast such a possibility; it emerged as an adaptive pattern under distinctive historical and cultural conditions, without consideration of which sex had more physical strength.

Third, considering human societies as a whole, men are more frequently assigned positions of power and authority in domestic, economic, and political arenas than women, but this generalization has been qualified by research (e.g., Sanday 1981). For example, earlier ethnographic accounts were sometimes biased in two ways: they described colonial situations in which women had lost power and authority formerly possessed in precolonial times, without recognition of their prior condition, and they reflected the views only of male informants, who sought to present women as powerless. Furthermore, it is now recognized that women often wield their power quietly in social contexts concealed from public view and that public ideologies emphasize the importance of men while underestimating the realities of female power—perhaps to protect vulnerable males from recognizing the threat. There are numerous ethnographic instances, brought to fuller light in recent years, in which women regularly occupied public positions as chiefs, kinship authorities, religious leaders, and even warriors. Even if women in their childbearing years are excluded from authoritative roles, postmenopausal women are often able to become leaders. It might also be mentioned that polyandry—the marital arrangement in which a woman marries more than one husband—though long thought to be limited to a few places in the Himalayas and Polynesia, has been documented in the peoples of central Nigeria (Levine and Sangree 1980).

Thus, though male dominance in social life is more prevalent than female dominance or egalitarian arrangements, the worldwide picture is not uniform, and within each society the relative status of women and men varies from one social domain to another (Quinn 1977; Sanday 1981).

Fourth, whatever the relationship of institutionalized gender roles and ideologies to gender-specific capacities in the human species, it is not like the close relationship between cultural patterns of communication and the human capacity for speech. In the case of speech, it can be confidently stated that every society has a language, with common features increasingly identified by linguists, and that speech is the primary means of interpersonal communication. Worldwide ethnographic investigation has *not* uncovered populations in which a significant minority of children fail to acquire the local language or where speech has been superseded by sign language in ordinary communication. In the case of institutionalized gender roles, however, only central tendencies among human societies can be related to male and female capacities, and we continue to learn of interesting exceptions, unpredictable from any theoretical premise except one that makes the realization of capacities heavily dependent on social and cultural conditions.

In other words, the more we know about human gender roles and differences through cross-cultural and historical research, the less support we can find for unqualified innatism or environmentalism. The more naive forms of sociobiology can be falsified by the fuller ethnographic data, but so can the proposition that any arrangement of gender roles is possible. That brings us to Margaret Mead's *Sex and Temperament in Three Primitive Societies,* which probably remains the most widely read anthropological book on the subject. When it was published in 1935, the book received unfavorable reviews in the major anthropological journals. Reviewers challenged the veracity of its ethnographic descriptions (Thurnwald 1936) and criticized its extreme environmentalism (Fortes 1936). These criticisms were well founded in the light of what we know today.

Sex roles vary within a narrower range than Mead claimed to have found in New Guinea. However, her message that gender constitutes an arena of great variability in human experience has borne up under empirical examination. The new evidence shows a wider variety of meanings attributed to being male and female than any existing theory could have generated. The basic contrasts of gender, including primary and secondary sexual characteristics, can be either elaborated or minimized in the symbolic representations of a culture; this is the dimension of cross-cultural variation. Meanings differ even among societies whose cultural idioms enhance the contrast between the sexes, like those of Mediterranean (including Hispanic) traditions and the people of Papua New Guinea. In both of these societies, for example, women may be symbols of dangerous sexuality, but Mediterranean cultures emphasize the purity of females while Papua New Guinea cultures represent them as impure and contaminating to men— with very different social consequences for women and families.

The most pervasive and unavoidable constraint on institutionalized gender roles is the woman's responsibility for the care of offspring. Reproduction is an obvious adaptive requirement, and there are clear limits on how completely fertility can be curtailed if a population is to survive. Theoretically, a wide variety of caretaking arrangements is possible. In fact, mothers almost everywhere take primary care of their own offspring, at least during the first 2 or 3 years of life. The assumption that women will provide the kind of care for their own infants that fosters infant survival and behavioral adaptation in the local context inevitably constrains the design of domestic life and gender roles.

The most notable exceptions to my statement that mothers usually care for their own offspring are the Israeli kibbutzim. Spiro (1958) provided a detailed ethnographic description of nonmaternal caretaking in one kibbutz. He returned 25 years later to find a widespread reassumption of traditional women's roles in the kibbutzim, with mothers much more deeply involved in the care of their own children. The strict feminist ideology of the founding mothers had been thrown

aside, even by many of the older mothers, in favor of almost una-
bashed endorsement of family-based child rearing. Spiro (1979), whose
own views had also changed in the interim from cultural environmentalism to a Freudian position that emphasizes "precultural"
aspects of personality development, interprets the kibbutz "counterrevolution" as the resurgence of a maternal motivation characteristic
of all women. He shows that the sabra mothers born on the kibbutz
and raised collectively under unisex conditions nonetheless showed
distinctively feminine orientations when he studied them as children
and preferred more traditionally feminine and maternal roles as adults.
Given the fact that the kibbutzim are not isolated communities, it is
difficult to prove that the counterrevolution in sex roles could not
have been caused by outside cultural influences or the persistent
influence of old models under new conditions of affluence.

Spiro's case for the precultural influence is a strong one, but it
should probably be seen as the beginning of a debate that will continue. Even as an unsettled issue, however, it indicates progress in
bringing comparative data to bear on a major question regarding the
development of women.

A serious challenge to existing conceptions of adolescent development, gender identity, and sexual object choice has been presented
by the New Guinea studies by Herdt (1981, 1982, 1984). In New Guinea,
a significant proportion of ethnic groups subject adolescent males to
initiation ceremonies that include homosexuality, or did earlier in
this century. Among the Sambia, with whom Herdt conducted fieldwork in the 1970s, boys typically spend 10 years in sexually active
relationships with men and boys and then marry and become husbands and fathers. Herdt's (1981) monograph portrays in rich detail
the cultural terms in which this transition is experienced.

What are we to make of the evidence? On the one hand, it can be
seen as supporting a universalist, innatist position regarding sexual
object choice because it shows that even prolonged, exclusively ho-
mosexual experience in adolescence need not deter males from reproduction in subsequent conjugal unions. On the other hand, it could
also be interpreted as support for a relativist, environmentalist position in which cultural symbols—idioms of masculinity, as Herdt
calls them—can make homosexuality seem normal and necessary, as
well as exciting, to a boy growing up in New Guinea, and despicably
abnormal or unimaginable to a boy growing up in Latin America,
the United States, and various other places. Both conclusions are
valid, yet the evidence calls for a more sophisticated analysis encompassing biological and cultural components.

## Conclusions

This brief overview indicates for the reader interested in psychiatric or developmental issues that anthropology continues to produce evidence, more detailed than before, concerning the experience of gender in diverse cultural settings. Recent anthropological data have given us a clearer picture of what is universal and what is variable in the social organization and cultural symbolization of gender in human societies. These data have also raised new questions, or revived old ones with a new complexity, concerning the plasticity of maternal behavior and sexuality under radically divergent conditions for human development. These questions, and the comparative psychosocial studies needed to answer them, will take their place on the research agenda for a deeper understanding of gender in the human species.

## References

Abu-Lughod L: Veiled Sentiments: Honor and Poetry in a Bedouin Society. Berkeley, CA, University of California Press, 1986

Fortes M: Review of sex and temperament in three primitive societies. Man 36:125–126, 1936

Herdt G: Guardians of the Flutes: Idioms of Masculinity. New York, McGraw-Hill, 1981

Herdt G (ed): Rituals of Manhood: Male Initiation in Papua New Guinea. Berkeley, CA, University of California Press, 1982

Herdt G (ed): Ritualized Homosexuality in Melanesia. Berkeley, CA, University of California Press, 1984

Levine N, Sangree W (eds): Women with many husbands: polyandrous alliance and marital flexibility in Africa and Asia. Journal of Comparative Family Studies 11 (entire issue), 1980

LeVine S: Mothers and Wives: Gusii Women of East Africa. Chicago, IL, University of Chicago Press, 1979

Mead M: Sex and Temperament in Three Primitive Societies. New York, Morrow, 1935

Quinn N: Anthropological studies on women's status. Annual Review of Anthropology 6:181–225, 1977

Sanday P: Female Power and Male Dominance: On the Origins of Sexual Inequality. New York, Cambridge University Press, 1981

Spiro M: Children of the Kibbutz. Cambridge, MA, Harvard University Press, 1958

Spiro M: Gender and Culture: Kibbutz Women Revisited. Durham, NC, Duke University Press, 1979

Thurnwald R: Review of sex and temperament in three primitive societies. American Anthropologist 38:663–667, 1936

Whiting B, Edwards C: A cross-cultural analysis of sex differences in the behavior of children aged three through eleven. J Soc Psychol 91:171–188, 1973

## Editors' Note

1. This chapter, in reviewing the range of societal solutions to gender roles and solutions to gender roles and the status of women and men illustrates not only the variation in patterns but also the variation of "normality." Dr. LeVine contrasts a universal capacity, such as the capacity for speech and its expression in language, with the case of institutionalized gender roles in which only their central tendency can be related to male or female capacities. He emphasizes the importance of both biological and cultural components to every gender pattern. New questions arise that can help the clinician to avoid absolute judgments and that illustrate the importance of considering the social context of a particular individual.

# Chapter 2

# Economic Perspectives on Work and Family Issues

## Hilda Kahne, Ph.D.

Women's changing values, activities, and roles over the past 20 years have set a sprightly course for the agenda of economic research on women. Although women have always worked, both in the home and in the marketplace, economic research on women in the 1940s and 1950s concentrated on their rapidly increasing *paid* work participation. With the growth of feminist interest in achieving economic equality for women, the research on paid work gradually became more focused on some disturbing aspects of women's work participation—the occupational segregation of women in the paid work that they do and the low level of their earnings compared with those of men. Some research attention was given to estimating the contribution of housewives to the gross national product (GNP), still omitted in measurement of our national accounts, and to the benefit loss that resulted from excluding that contribution in computing the level of social security benefits. But the central focus of economists' interests remained primarily with paid work, advancing both economic theory relating to women's experience and policy proposals to make women's opportunities, work environments, and economic rewards more equitable.

In recent years, it has become increasingly evident—to economists no less than to other social scientists—that the issues surrounding women's paid work cannot be divorced from family concerns. Changing marital and fertility patterns, and continuing pressure on the scarce resource of time facing women who must accommodate both work and family demands, have broad social science implications not limited to any one discipline. The increasing need for cross-disciplinary exchange about work and family concerns was reflected in the establishment of an interdisciplinary *Annual Review of Women and Work*, now in its third edition (Gutek et al. 1988), and a first Lace Professorship of Families, Change, and Society, established in 1986 at Wheaton College to stimulate and coordinate interdisciplinary teaching and research on family issues. This forum represents another way of furthering this evolving cross-disciplinary tradition that stimulates discussion of gender differences that relate to work and family issues.

In this chapter, I discuss findings in three policy-related economic research areas, each growing out of changes in women's lives during the past 20 years and each having cross-disciplinary implications. I will not elaborate the economic theories of our discipline in this area, although they too have experienced an evolution, sometimes providing a useful context for interpreting data and sometimes divorced from or lagging behind what we know to be the reality of women's lives.

## Women's Paid Work Participation—Recent Gains and Gender Differences

What do we know about paid work participation of women (that is, the percentage of women in the civilian labor force) and their employment experience?

The participation of women in the paid labor force has been rising since the turn of the century. But the rate of increase of that growth since World War II has been so dramatic that one labor expert, Eli Ginzberg, has described it as the single most dramatic event of the twentieth century. Between 1972 and 1983, women accounted for two-thirds of the growth of the labor force. Between 1950 and 1989, when male labor force participation rates fell from 86% to 76% because of extended schooling and earlier retirement (although there was no change in paid work rates in the prime adult years), the labor force participation rate of women rose from 34% to 58%. In the early post–World War II period, the rising rate was strongly influenced by the entry of women aged 45–64 years after their children had grown. Since 1960, the dramatic growth has been among married women, most recently among those with young children. In 1959, about one-third of all women and only 12% of women with young children were in the labor force. By 1988, however, participation rates of all women and of married women—whether or not they had preschool children—were all over 50%: 56% of all married women and 50% of married women with children under age 6 were in the labor force (U.S. Department of Labor 1988). Between 1952 and 1982, the labor force participation rate of all women rose 50%, doubled for married women, and tripled for married women with young children. It is expected that while men's work rates will continue to decline in the years ahead, those of women will continue to grow, although the pace will be slower than in the past. By 2000, perhaps 47% of all workers will be women and women's labor force participation rate will be about 63% (Fullerton 1989). That is what is meant by saying that feminization of the labor force has taken place. It is clear that the sex composition of the labor force in the future will be markedly different from that of the past.

A number of economic and noneconomic factors have combined to bring about this rise in women's paid work. Reasons include both an increased demand for women workers to fill the growing numbers of service and other "female-typed" job openings that have come with changing occupational structures, and an increased supply of workers due to rising aspirations and desire for autonomy, increased education, and a need for income to meet family needs or to maintain a standard of living. Women seem to respond more strongly to what economists call the substitution effect, exchanging paid work hours for leisure as their own earnings rise (leisure becoming more expensive), rather than to the countervailing income effect, in which the motivation is to gain more leisure by working fewer hours, made possible by a rising family income. Whatever the causes, we now live in a society where both adult women and men are more apt to be employed than not employed. This is a major change that makes the effect of paid work on people's lives extremely important. Moreover, in 1988, 55% of married women with children under age 3 years were in the labor force. These mothers represent the fastest growing segment of the labor force today. This explains why parental leave and child care are two of the most important policy issues today.

The contribution of women's earnings to family income is one economic aspect of this situation. Working women contribute about 30% to family income overall, 40% when they work full-time year-round (U.S. Department of Commerce 1984). Another important aspect is the effect of paid work on work-family conflict, an effect that can be different for women than for men. Joseph Pleck and colleagues (1980), for example, report that men experience tension over the length of their work hours; women more often report work schedule incompatibilities with other responsibilities and fatigue and irritability that impinge on the harmony of family life. No one has to be convinced that paid work is a mixed blessing. We need to spell out the range of effects and their interrelationships and intensity for women and for men, so that developed policies can lessen the negative and reinforce the positive influences of paid work on people's lives.

One negative aspect of labor force attachment comes when unemployment removes the source of economic security that has come to be relied on. Unemployment means for the individual a loss of income as well as a psychological loss of community and social experience. Marie Jahoda explored these consequences of unemployment in 1933 and reflected about them again in 1982 when she wrote that among the several kinds of benefits provided by paid work are "the imposition of a time structure, the enlargement of the scope of social experience into areas less emotionally charged than family life, participation in a collective purpose or effort, the assignment by virtue of employment of status and identity and required regular activity" (p. 59). Harvey Brenner found, in analysis of data of a national population sample in the early 1970s, a rise in mortality, suicide rate, cardiovascular death, and mental breakdown accompanying unemployment (Brenner 1982, 1984). Liem and Rayman (1981, 1982), in a more qualitative study of the effects of unemployment stress on unemployed men and their spouses in several New England areas, found an increase in depression, anxiety, and hostility resulting in more marriage breakups and more parent-child conflict and child abuse. Unemployment leads to both noneconomic and economic sources of stress. Both must be dealt with in countering the effects of unemployment.

In economic terms, it has been found that unemployment, like labor force participation, has different implications for women and for men. Miller (1986) noted that deindustrialization and employment in gender-typed occupations have led in recent years to lower cyclical unemployment rates for women than for men. On the other hand, women constitute three-fifths of the 1.6 million discouraged unemployed workers who want a job but who are not counted as unemployed because they have left the labor force thinking that no jobs are available. Social policies that respond to needs of unemployed women may require different and more intensive job-search assistance than for men to counter the absence of networks, the larger turnover rates, and the different kinds of job training needed to expand occupational options. New forms of income supports could allocate funds to both training and family care when routine family needs are already provided by another family income.

The specific characteristics of women's occupational distribution and earnings provide further evidence of the distinctiveness of their labor market experience. For one thing, women work in fewer occupations than do men. About one-fourth of all women's employment is concentrated among just 22 of the 500 U.S. Census Bureau's occupational categories; men's employment is largely divided among the rest. Women also work in different occupations than men. Over one-half of the 500 occupational categories in the 1980 U.S. Census included either more than 80% female workers or 80% male workers (Reskin and Hartmann 1986). Women cluster in clerical work (in which one-third of women work) and low-level service and trade occupations. Moreover, even within the same occupation, women work in different departments from men: in health care, women work as food handlers and men work as orderlies; women sales personnel work in department stores, men in sales are more likely to be found in automobile dealerships.

Gender desegregation has far to go, especially in areas such as skilled craft work where the pay is relatively high (Reskin 1984). In the 1970s, there was some lessening of segregation, due partly to the enforcement of affirmative action legislation (Beller 1984; Beller and Han 1984), partly to the increasing number of women who chose nontraditional training and occupational directions, and partly to the side effects of recession, where some men were forced to accept less desirable jobs formerly thought of as "female" occupations. Between 1970 and 1980, the percentage of women in managerial and skilled craft work increased relative to their increase in the labor force as a whole, while the percentage of women in lower-paying service jobs fell. At the same time, desegregation of occupations was spurred by the fact that men moved into some "female" occupations, for example, the secretarial and nursing fields. The improvements showed up particularly for new and recent labor market entrants and those in white-collar occupations. But although an index of segregation in the 1970s declined at an average annual rate almost three times as large as that during the 1960s, it still was almost 62% in 1981 (68% in 1972). This means that about three of five workers of one sex would have to be redistributed among occupations for the occupational distribution to reach complete equality between the sexes. The rate of segregation decline has been much reduced in the 1980s, and there is even some evidence of resegregation (Blau and Ferber 1986b).

What does the future hold? Some improvement is likely as women enter nontraditional jobs and growth occurs in occupations that are relatively desegregated (e.g., computer jobs). On the other hand, the number of skilled craft workers, heavily male, is expected to show moderate growth; if this is not to cause a slowdown in desegregation, social policy must also foster women's entrance into these areas (Beller 1984). We are still far from being able to say that work opportunities for women and men are approaching equality.

Occupational desegregation has important implications for employment mobility and flexibility, career progress, and earnings. But no less important than these economic aspects of work are the effects of work environment (including those that are nontraditional) on women (see, e.g., Kanter 1977; O'Farrell and Harlan 1984), and the effect changing gender roles can have in influencing that environment. Devising techniques for recruiting and training women for nontraditional jobs and designing ways of helping women gain a sense of competence and confidence in unfamiliar and often uncordial settings are not basic, perhaps, to traditional economic inquiry, but the consequences of such programs certainly are fundamental to an improved economic functioning of the labor market (O'Farrell 1988).

A number of economists hold the view that because occupational segregation leads to "crowding," which lowers the marginal productivity of women workers, it is a causal factor of the earnings gap between women and men. Women's median weekly earnings hovered between 60% and 63% of men's earnings between 1967 and 1980 and rose to 70% in 1986. It appears that the earnings discrepancy is diminishing, although the differential continues to be large (Blau and Ferber 1986a, 1986b).

Over the years, a number of studies sought to explain the large gap between earnings of women and men. Their findings suggest that less than half of the gross earnings differential of about 40% can be attributed to factors associated with productivity differences between individuals or jobs (e.g., job skills, years of schooling, or years of experience). The large unexplained residual is probably caused by discriminatory and socialization factors, including occupational segregation, which plays a significant role in depressing women's wages (Reskin and Hartmann 1986).

Legislative policy in the 1960s sought improvement in women's relative earnings through an affirmative action policy that mandated equal pay for substantially equal jobs. But as it became clear that women and men worked in different jobs, which precluded the effectiveness of such a standard, an extension of affirmative action was developed in the form of a comparable-worth philosophy. In this view, women's earnings are low not necessarily because of intentional discrimination by an individual employer, but because women traditionally do work that is undervalued by society. A policy of comparable worth, supported by groups seeking improved pay equity, would raise earnings in occupations where women traditionally work by evaluating and comparing characteristics of the job—job skills, effort, responsibility, and working conditions—and raising women's wages to match those of men whose jobs have similar qualities. In the United States, such a policy is still largely limited to public sector jobs or to enterprises in specific occupations, with wages adjusted through collective bargaining. In Canada and some European countries, on the other hand, the concept is broadly applied across the entire range of work situations, with considerable popularity and efficiency. Comparable worth has been identified as "the civil rights issue of the eighties." Despite complexity in its application, comparable worth is increasingly being used to rationalize wages within an enterprise and upgrade women's wages to match those of men's jobs with similar characteristics (Aaron and Laugy 1986; Hartmann 1985; Remick 1984).

## Changing Family Structures and Consequences

Just as the dynamic movement of paid work raises a host of new research issues affecting women's lives, so too do changing longevity, marital and fertility patterns, and gender roles. The longevity of women (which is not only increasing, but increasing more rapidly than that of men), the increased proportion of women who postpone first marriages, the increasing prevalence of two-earner marriages (which now affect over three-fifths of married-couple families), the high frequency of divorce, and the increase in teen and preteen pregnancy all have implications for life-cycle rhythms and life consequences that encompass, and extend beyond, economic interpretation. A variety of issues could illustrate multidisciplinary research interests in this area. I will focus remarks on the economic status and needs of female family heads.

About 17% of all families (10.5 million families in March 1988) are headed by women. Since 1970, this type of family has increased four times as fast as all families (Johnson and Waldman 1983; U.S. Census Bureau 1985). Forty-four percent of black families compared to 13% of white families are maintained by women. A major factor in the rapid growth of woman-headed families has been the large number of marriages of the baby boom generation and subsequent higher divorce rates, which today are equivalent to one divorce for every two first marriages. Also contributing to this growth, particularly since the 1970s, has been the sharp rise in childbearing among single women, especially teenagers

(U.S. Commission on Civil Rights 1983), among whom the pregnancy rate is twice that of Britain and four times that of Canada. One of every two teenage mothers is unmarried. Unlike the period of the 1970s, when over two-fifths of women maintaining families were widowed, in 1987, 64% of females maintaining families were separated or divorced and another 30% had never been married. Because they have lower educational levels and fewer skills, female family heads often work in less skilled and lower paid occupations—as typists, cashiers, office and hotel cleaners, waitresses, and nurses' aides (Sarris 1984). Compared with married-couple families, fewer women who head families live in multiple-earner families (56% versus 30%). Their unemployment rates are higher than those of husband and wife families. The situation is particularly devastating in black female-headed families, where more children, lower labor force participation rates, lower median earnings, and higher unemployment rates prevail.

I need hardly spell out the kinds of distress that accompany the too early curtailing of life's options and the effect of overwhelming family responsibility without the support of adequate coping skills and family or social support. Research documents the considerable movement in and out of these circumstances, the plight of single parents, including children who are mothers, and the needs of their children (Duncan 1984). The loneliness of single mothers who head families, their lack of a sense of self-worth, and the practical problems of child and after-school care are all examples of difficult life problems that confront these women.

In economic terms, female family heads constitute a category contributing to a frightening new societal problem—the "feminization of poverty." Although 60% of female family heads are in the labor force, one in three families maintained by women is in poverty, and almost 50% of families in poverty are maintained by women. Even with full-time work, about 6.2% of families headed by women were below the poverty level in 1983. These women need a range of family and work-related supports: job training, job search assistance, work schedule flexibility, child care, and parental leave, none of which is part of our national social legislation. Such programs would benefit not only women but also the children of our society, half of whom are expected to live with a single parent for some period during their growing years. Their long-term well-being is becoming a matter of increasing social concern.

## Part-time Work—Needs and Benefits

Changing aspirations of women, the increasing proportion of women committed to continuous paid work throughout adulthood, changing marital patterns that result in a need for economic autonomy, and home, child, and elder care responsibilities provide the foundation for a third policy-related economic issue—part-time work. This work structure has particular meaning for women who must have work schedule flexibility to meet the heavy combined demands of work and home (Kahne 1985; Kahne, in press). "New concept part-time work" includes prorated full-time wage and equivalent fringe benefits, together with a permanent attachment to the job and a potential for career advancement, and provides one form of flexibility. For men, part-time work is often identified with young workers who also attend school or with older workers who stand to benefit from a gradual phasing into retirement. For women, however, the need for reduced-hour work schedules can occur throughout life. About 25% of married and single women and 13% of divorced women work part-time schedules even though the pay is often low and not equivalent to that for full-time work, and fringe benefits are often absent.

Since the 1940s, about 40% of the dramatic increase in the number of working women has been in part-time employment. Studies show that there is no single way that part-time work is used. Sometimes it is an alternative to full-time work; for other women it serves as an alternative to not working. But very few women use it as a transition into the labor market and gradually into full-time work (Blank 1988). In recent years there has been a gradual increase in "New Concept part-time work" in the form of work sharing, job sharing, and regular part-time. What is interesting—and surprising—is that there has not been a stronger movement toward expansion of New Concept part-time work, even with growing evidence of both cost-saving benefits for employers and schedule flexibility benefits for workers (Kahne 1985). Despite demographic changes in labor force composition and in occupational and industrial trends that are conducive to the introduction of part-time work, changes in values, roles, and activities of individuals have occurred much more easily than have the needed changes in societal institutions.

Research in several social science disciplines relates to work schedule pressures and the issues relevant to their restructuring. Studies have identified a number of work-family dilemmas that two-worker families must confront (Moen 1982): the different time demands on husbands and wives to fulfill paid work and family care needs (Pleck 1985), and the different kinds of tensions and family-work conflicts that husbands and wives face (Pleck et al. 1980). Although "role overload" for wives in terms of total family and work hours is less important an issue than it was in the 1960s and early 1970s, wives still spend more hours than husbands in family care. Between 1965 and

1981, for example, husbands' time spent in housework and child care rose from about 20% to 30% of time spent by the couple in such activities (Juster and Stafford 1986)—a marked improvement, but far from an equal share. Women also frequently do the less pleasurable family care and household tasks and assume administrative responsibility for ensuring that the needs are met. This proportion is probably continuing to increase, but very slowly.

Despite the fact that half of all women with children under age 3 and 70% of women whose youngest child is 6–13 years old are in the labor force, socially supported child care is extremely limited and, when provided, often is concerned with providing information rather than service. With respect to the elderly, one national study of primary caregivers of moderately to severely impaired elderly persons living in the household of the caretaker estimated that 70% of the caregivers were women. About 50% of female caregivers under age 65 also had paid jobs (Soldo 1980). Demographic projections suggest that the number of elderly persons may double between 1980 and 2020 and the number of the frail elderly (ages 85 and over) may triple. Access to reduced work hours for women is critically important in periods of their lives when family care responsibilities must take precedence over full-time paid work. Unless some work-hour flexibility is introduced, women will continue to be required to make painful choices, frequently deciding to leave the labor market during periods when they must devote energies to home needs. When they do this, not only earnings but also career progression and retirement pensions will suffer, and society will lose the productive contribution of valuable human resources.

Hard choices of this kind need not be necessary. Studies suggest that part-time work in a wide range of occupations is both possible and efficient (Kahne 1985). Work weeks of less than 40 hours (regular part-time, job sharing, phased retirement, work sharing) exist in both blue-collar and white-collar jobs. These forms have been successfully applied to highly professional occupations where employees work autonomously, and to semiskilled manufacturing assembly work where interaction among workers and between workers and machines is essential. Studies show that reduced-hour work can result in benefits of increased productivity, access to valued human resources, and cost savings in the form of reduced absenteeism and labor turnover and less overtime pay (Kahne 1985). With respect to the problem of those fringe-benefit costs that cannot be prorated, enterprises and worker representatives have developed techniques for "cashing out" benefits, sharing costs, or limiting the employer's financial commitment through such techniques as "cafeteria" benefits. New Concept part-time work, thus, can offer improved efficiency to employers as well as the benefit of "time" for women in critical periods of their lives. This kind of work schedule needs more visibility and should be available without penalty to women or men.

Part-time work illustrates a larger multidisciplinary subject having to do with the workplace—work organization, remuneration, and environment—that affects women's lives. Work motivation, job environment, worker output, wages, fringe benefits, and parental leave all are part of research on labor economics and research in other areas concerned with the well-being of individuals and the quality of their work lives and with changes in work organization and productivity that improve the competitive position of American industry. The beneficial changes in the work environment that result from the availability of a broader range of work schedule alternatives provide only one example of how the workplace is—and must continue to be—improved in response to the increasing feminization of the labor force.

## Conclusion

None of us need the evidence of research to tell us that work and family issues for women are inextricably intertwined and that they also have implications for the men with whom women share their lives. But research can help us understand what is happening with changing gender roles and the increasing scarcity of time for their expression, as well as with the consequences and policy implications of these changes for society.

In this chapter, I discussed some of the research issues concerning women's paid work and family roles with which economics is concerned—labor force participation, unemployment, occupational and earnings experience, economic status of female family heads—emphasizing the cross-disciplinary research linkages of each issue. Recognizing that changes in worker characteristics and activities inevitably have repercussions for work environments and social structures, I also explored the experience of "New Concept part-time work" scheduling (paying prorated wages and at least some fringe benefits) as one aspect of the institution of the workplace that would benefit from reevaluation and adaptation to the new life-styles.

The complexity of evolutionary change—for both individuals and institutions—inevitably blurs disciplinary lines and provides common themes for consideration by social scientists. The more we talk and work together, the more complete will be our understanding of the rapid social changes that we are experiencing. Our common efforts to interpret that experience, however, can go further than this. They can help to ensure that policy responses to the inevitable changes not only move us, but move us in positive directions.

## References

Aaron HJ, Laugy CM: The Comparable Worth Controversy. Washington, DC, Brookings Institution, 1986

Beller A: Trends in occupational segregation by sex and race, 1960–81, in Sex Segregation in the Workplace: Trends, Explanations, Remedies. Edited by Reskin BF. Washington, DC, National Academy Press, 1984, pp 11–26

Beller A, Han KK: Occupational sex segregation: prospects for the 1980s, in Sex Segregation in the Workplace: Trends, Explanations, Remedies. Edited by Reskin BF. Washington, DC, National Academy Press, 1984, pp 91–114

Blank R: The role of part-time work in women's labor market choices over time. Presented at the American Economic Association meeting, Dec 1988

Blau FD, Ferber MA: The Economics of Women, Men, and Work. Englewood Cliffs, NJ, Prentice-Hall, 1986a

Blau FD, Ferber MA: Women's progress in the labor market: should we rest on our laurels? Proceedings of the 39th Annual Proceedings of the Industrial Relations Research Association, 1986b

Brenner H: Assessing the social costs of national unemployment rates for the older population, in The Unemployment Crisis Facing Older Americans. U.S. Select Committee on Aging, Hearings, 97th Congress, 2nd Session, Oct 8, 1982, pp 45–48

Brenner H: Estimating the effects of economic change on national health and social well being. Study prepared for the use of the Subcommittee on Economic Goals and Intergovernmental Policy, Joint Economic Committee, U.S. Congress, 98th Congress, 2nd Session, June 15, 1984

Duncan GJ: Years of Poverty, Years of Plenty. Ann Arbor, MI, Institute for Social Research, University of Michigan, 1984

Fullerton HN Jr: New labor force projections, spanning 1988 to 2000. Monthly Labor Review 112:3–12, 1989

Gutek B, Stromberg A, Larwood L (eds): Women and Work—An Annual Review, Vol 3. Beverly Hills, CA, Sage, 1988

Hartmann H (ed): Comparable Worth: New Dimensions for Research. Washington, DC, National Academy Press, 1985

Jahoda M: Employment and Unemployment: A Social Psychological Analysis. Cambridge, England, Cambridge University Press, 1982

Jahoda M, Lazarsfeld P, Zeisel H: Marienthal: The Sociography of an Unemployed Community. Chicago, IL, Aldine-Atherton, 1933

Johnson BL, Waldman E: Most women who maintain families receive poor
job market returns. Monthly Labor Review 106:30–34, 1983

Juster FT, Stafford F (eds): Time, Goods and Well Being. Ann Arbor, MI,
Institute for Social Research, University of Michigan, 1986

Kahne H: Reconceiving Part-time Work: New Perspectives for Older Workers and Women. Totawa, NJ, Rowman & Allanheld, 1985

Kahne H: Part-time work: a hope and a peril, in Part-time Work: Opportunity or Dead End. Edited by Lundy K, Warme B. New York, Praeger
(in press)

Kanter R: Men and Women of the Corporation. New York, Basic Books,
1977

Liem R: Employment and mental health implications for human services
policy. Policy Studies Journal 10:350–364, 1981

Liem R, Rayman P: Health and social costs of unemployment: research
and policy considerations. Am Psychol 37:116–173, 1982

Miller J: Women's unemployment patterns in post-war business cycles:
the gender segregation of work and deindustrialization. Paper presented at Eastern Economics Association Meeting, Philadelphia, PA,
April 1986

Moen P: The two provider family: problems and potentials, in Nontraditional Families: Parenting and Child Development. Edited by Lamb
ME. Hillsdale, NJ, Lawrence Erlbaum, 1982

O'Farrell B: Women in blue collar occupations, traditional and nontra-
ditional, in Women Working: Theories and Facts in Perspective, 2nd
Edition. Edited by Stromberg AH, Harkness S. Mountain View, CA,
Mayfield, 1987

O'Farrell B, Harlan SH: Job integration strategies: today's programs and
tomorrow's needs, in Sex Segregation in the Workplace: Trends, Explanations, Remedies. Edited by Reskin BF. Washington, DC, National
Academy Press, 1984, pp 267–291

Pleck JH: Working Wives/Working Husbands. Beverly Hills, CA, Sage, 1985

Pleck JH, Staines GL, Lang L: Conflicts between work and family life.
Monthly Labor Review 103:29–32, 1980

Remick H (ed): Comparable Worth and Wage Discrimination: Technical
Possibilities and Political Realities. Philadelphia, PA, Temple University Press, 1984

Reskin BF (ed): Sex Segregation in the Workplace: Trends, Explanations,
Remedies. Washington, DC, National Academy Press, 1984

Reskin BF, Hartmann HI (eds): Women's Work, Men's Work: Sex Segregation on the Job. Washington, DC, National Academy Press, 1986

Sarris R: The 1981 Omnibus Reconciliation Act and Aid for Families With
Dependent Children. Ann Arbor, MI, Institute for Social Research,
University of Michigan, 1984

Soldo BJ: Family caregiving and the elderly: prevalence and variations. Final Report. Washington, DC, Kennedy Institute, Georgetown University, 1980

U.S. Census Bureau: Population profile of the United States. Current Population Reports, Special Studies, Series P-23, No 145, 1985

U.S. Commission on Civil Rights: A Growing Crisis: Disadvantaged Women and Their Children. May 1983

U.S. Department of Commerce: Earnings in 1981 of married couple families by selected characteristics of husbands and wives. Current Population Reports, Special Studies, Series P-23, No 133, March 1984

U.S. Department of Labor, Bureau of Labor Statistics: News (Labor Force Participation and Marital Status). Sept 7, 1988

*Chapter 3*

# A Review of Gender Differences in Brain and Behavior

**Malkah T. Notman, M.D.**
**Carol C. Nadelson, M.D.**

In this chapter, we summarize some of the research on gender differences in brain structure and functioning and related topics that have appeared in the neurology and psychology literature. This is not an exhaustive or even a comprehensive summary of this vast and complex area, but it will orient the reader to the current state of the field.

It is clear that whatever innate biologically determined differences exist between men and women, their expression in behavior, talent, or ability is profoundly affected by cultural patterns and socialization. As Dr. Gilligan notes in Chapter 10, there is no one universal human culture, but an enormous range of cultural expression among different groups. Within each group are a man's culture and a woman's culture; the experiences of each gender are different. A number of studies, such as those on the influence of prenatal factors and early development experiences, have described the reciprocal influences of biological and experiential factors. The implications of these data for understanding the lives of women and men and the concepts of normality and psychopathology are substantial.

Nevertheless, the pursuit of what are considered by some to be the "true" or biological gender differences in neurological structure and function remains active. Drs. Russo and Bleier, in Chapters 5 and 6, respectively, discuss some of the problems with this work. It is useful to review here some of the major ideas and findings that enter into this controversy.

Restak (1979) reviews data on differences between men and women attributed to the brain. In quotes from two well-known writers, he illustrates two different perspectives:

> Reasoning is of feminine nature; it can give only after it has received.
> Schopenhauer, *The World as Will and Representation*,
> translated 1966

> There is no female mind. The brain is not an organ of sex. As well speak of the female liver.
> Charlotte Perkins Gillman, *Women in Economics*, 1898

Restak also reminds the reader that gender differences are meaningful on a statistical rather than an individual basis. He notes that there are several areas where brain gender differences have been found to exist. He summarizes studies confirming that women favor a "communicative mode" in gaining knowledge about the world and in dealing with others. For example, from birth, female infants are more sensitive to sounds, particularly the mother's voice. As babies, females orient more to tone than males and are more startled by loud noises. They maintain enhanced hearing throughout life.

In other sensory skills, girls have also been shown to do better than boys: girls have increased skin sensitivity, they are more proficient in fine motor performance, and they do better at rapid sequential movements. Girls are also thought to be at an advantage in tasks that require organizing data in sequence. Boys are different in that different stimuli attract their attention; females are more attentive to social contexts such as faces, speech patterns, and tones of voice. Female infants can speak sooner, and, throughout life, women do better on a number of measures of linguistic ability. Restak states that boys, however, show an early superiority in visual acuity. In his review, Restak also reflects the stereotype of male and female differences, and does not question the design or validity of the studies he quotes.

Recent findings regarding lateralization of the brain will enable further understanding of these differences. "In most right-handed individuals the left hemisphere is specialized for language and related serial processing of information, whereas the right hemisphere is specialized for a variety of nonverbal processes, including three-dimensional visualization, mental rotation, face recognition, and understanding the meaning of facial expressions" (Kelly 1985, p. 781).

The research data related to this information come from many sources. Hemispheric lateralization—the difference in the two hemispheres of the brain in their capabilities such as speech—was established in the late 1960s and 1970s (Geschwind and Levitsky 1968). McGuiness found that boys are more curious in exploring the environment and in being able to mentally rotate or fold an object (Restak 1979). To support the idea that the latter ability is a biologically determined difference, Restak cited electroencephalographic data documenting a difference in response between boys and girls in performing a test consisting of presenting an irregular piece of paper, used for the rotating and folding tests, to the right or the left visual field. "In boys, the fastest response always follows the presentation to the left visual fields (right hemisphere)," while girls do their best when the material is presented to the right visual field, "indicating that they use their left hemisphere for both visual spatial processing and verbal tasks" (Restak 1979, p. 200). Observed differences between males and females in math and verbal abilities have stimulated explanations based on the extent of lateralization of the brain in males compared with females. Males have been considered to have greater lateralization.

The generally accepted conclusion, that girls use the left hemisphere for both verbal and spatial processing, is the basis of a theory proposed by psychologist Jerre Levy (1972, 1977) that there is a process of "log jamming" in women in which "the use of words to solve a spatial problem results in slow, incorrect or absent responses because of a kind of interference. Males, who are specialized for visual functions in the right hemisphere, are generally observed to be more proficient in visual-spatial tasks" (Restak 1979, pp. 200–201).

Restak (1979) supports this view by citing a number of other gender differences in performance, including performance on the Wechsler Adult Intelligence Scale. He also cites tests of field dependence and independence that measured the ability to carry out a test procedure while ignoring irrelevant and extraneous stimuli.

A number of researchers have discussed sex differences in patterns of cognitive asymmetry and in rates of maturation of cognitive functions in the two hemispheres (Kelly 1985; Kupferman 1985; Witelson 1976, 1978, 1985a, 1986). In one series of studies, females were shown to be more "field dependent" than males, meaning that they tend to see stimuli in context rather than independent of context. The generalizability of these findings regarding field dependence beyond the specific test situation has been questioned and is not now universally accepted, but it has been argued clinically that this finding is consistent with women's greater involvement in relationships and in their concerns about separation (Henley 1985). However, clinical experience may have influenced the readiness for many investigators and clinicians to generalize from the limited psychological tests. The waxing and waning of ideas about field dependence and its applications as a theory have been discussed in a review of these studies and their current status by Henley (1985).

One can also consider the well-known studies of individuals whose genetic sex is different than their manifest phenotypic sex because of abnormalities affecting the utilization of the circulating androgens. In the condition known as "testicular feminization," or "androgen insensitivity syndrome," the individual is genotypically male and phenotypically female. That is, the genitals appear female grossly because of failure to respond to the further differentiation ordinarily stimulated by the fetal circulating male hormones. Individuals with this disorder who were raised as females have been found to have a predominantly feminine style despite the male chromosomal pattern; those individuals raised as males developed a predominantly masculine style (Money and Ehrhardt 1972). This finding supports the view that resulting male-female differences are strongly influenced by socialization and are the product of interactions between the biological and the experiential processes.

Another perspective on the nature of biological processes is provided by Kandel, who argues that the distinction between the biological, or structural, basis of behavior and the experiential, or functional, is artificial. He reviews many studies and concludes that

> Everyday events—sensory stimulation, deprivation, and learning—have profound biological consequences, causing an effective disruption of synaptic connections under some circumstances, and a reactivation of connections under others. It therefore is incorrect to imply that certain diseases (organic diseases) affect mentation by producing biological changes in the brain, whereas other diseases (functional diseases) do not. All mental processes are biological and any alteration in these processes is organic. . . . Even in the most socially determined mental disturbances, the end result is biological, since it is the activity of the brain that is being modified. Insofar as social intervention, such as psychotherapy or counseling, works, it must work by acting on the brain, quite likely on the connections between nerve cells. (Kandel 1985, p. 831)

If one extends Kandel's position, the search for the biological origin of gender differences, often considered the "bedrock," may be less important than a focus on the interaction of biological and experiential processes.

Witelson (1976, 1978, 1985a, 1985b, 1986) has been a proponent of the existence of biological genetic differences in aptitudes and motivation between men and women. In discussing the differences in math scores between 7th and 8th grade boys and girls, she states that "the superior performance in mathematics which is present in childhood may be a result of 'both endogenous and exogenous variables.' In view of current neurological findings such results certainly warrant the hypothesis of the operation of some natural factor" (Witelson 1985b, p. 54). The "natural factor" is understood to be a biological one.

Witelson has also pointed to the importance of hormonal effects in gender differences. She recognizes that the biological factors are easier to study than the environmental causes of some behaviors where there are evident gender differences. To do the kind of environmental manipulation needed to demonstrate that a sociological factor affects a reported sex difference in behavior is difficult (Witelson 1986).

One of Witelson's widely quoted studies concerns the relative participation of the two cerebral hemispheres in spatial processing (Witelson 1976). In one study, she tested boys and girls between ages 6 and 13 and gave them two different meaningless shapes to palpate simultaneously, out of sight and one in each hand, for a 10-second period. They were then asked to identify the objects from pictures. In describing this study she writes (p. 425).

> The test has two crucial features. 1. It requires tactile shape discrimination which, in adults, depends mainly on the right hemisphere. 2. Different stimuli are presented simultaneously. . . . It was hoped that this procedure would produce competition in the nervous system . . . such that any superiority of the right hemisphere for the required cognitive processing would be reflected in superior perception of the contra-lateral (left) hand stimuli.

Witelson found that this was true only for boys, who "performed in a manner consistent with right hemisphere specialization as early as six years old," regardless of their level of proficiency, which largely overlapped that of girls. Girls showed evidence of bilateral representation (no clear hand superiority) until the age of 13, "suggesting that boys have greater hemispheric specialization and that there is a sexual dimorphism in the neural organization related to cognition for an extended period of development" (Witelson 1976, p. 425).

Witelson concludes,

> The superiority of males to females on many, although not all, spatial tests may be related to the hypothesized neural dimorphism. Spatial

ability seems to be related to sex chromosomes and testosterone levels. Such genetic and hormonal factors may cause the neural dimorphism in the sexes which in turn may underlie the sex differences in spatial ability. (p. 426)

She then adds:

If the right hemisphere in girls is not specialized for a particular cognitive function, then the brain of young females, particularly the right hemisphere, may have greater plasticity for a longer period than that of males. Thus, language functions may transfer more readily to the right hemisphere in females than in males following early damage to the left hemisphere; in fact, for patients with early lesions, women show less impairment than men on verbal tasks after neurosurgical removal of left hemisphere tissue at maturity.

Greater plasticity of the young female brain also suggests that females may have a lower incidence of developmental disorders associated with possible left hemisphere dysfunction and for which greater plasticity of the right hemisphere might be advantageous. Males do have a higher incidence than females of developmental dyslexia, developmental aphasia and infantile autism, all of which have language deficits as a predominant symptom. (Witelson 1976, p. 426)[1]

Kelly (1985) discusses the wide range of behavior that is influenced by sex differences in central nervous system organization. He raises questions about the types of behavior that might be influenced by sex differences in the cellular organization of the brain, and to what "extent sexually differentiated neural organization and its consequent behavioral biases might be influenced by environmental events" in the life span of the individual (p. 780). He cites several lines of evidence that the perinatal hormonal environment influences behaviors that might extend well beyond reproductive behaviors.

## Developmental Framework

A developmental framework is also important in understanding these findings. Kelly cites work with primates on the effects of exposure to prenatal hormones. He refers to McEwen's work demonstrating that the frontal cerebral cortex of the monkey is sexually dimorphic in its rate of development, possibly related to the existence of the steroid-sensitive neurons in the frontal cortex of rats. "These receptor sites, demonstrable only in infancy, have been reported by McEwen to disappear by puberty" (Kelly 1985, p. 781). The developmental timing of the maturation of various structures and the interrelationship to the presence of hormones at a given time are thus the complex ways by which genetic differences, which control the amount and kinds of prenatal hormones, can influence neural organization.

Kelly states, "Although our understanding of sex differences in human neural organization is still limited, it seems clear that the range of gender-typical behavioral biases that may be related to perinatal events are quite broad and that biologically-based sex differences are not limited to reproductive behavior" (Kelly 1985, p. 782). He also stresses the importance of learning and the flexibility of most behaviors. It is clear that this is an area for ongoing research and careful review because biologically based sex differences have been taken to mean differences in ability.

## Gender Differences in Sensations

Another interesting area of study has been gender differences in sensory functions. In this field, the research is also uneven. In a review article, Velle (1987) summarizes the data on gender differences in sensory functions. Although there are greater variations among individuals than between men and women in many functions, some gender differences do emerge consistently in taste, smell, hearing, vision, and skin sensations.

In relation to taste, Velle states (p. 491), "when the sexes were compared, no significant differences in sensitivity were observed up to the age of 40. After 40, however, sex differences became increasingly greater, women retaining higher sensitivity than men for all four [taste] substances tested." In a number of studies the sensitivity of the organs to the substances tested is higher, on average, in women than in men. The basis of these gender differences in taste function is unknown. Velle reports, however, that a number of studies strongly suggest that sex hormones influence sensitivity to taste as well as taste preferences.

Sensitivity to smell also appears to be different for men and women. Velle states (p. 495), "a number of well-planned and convincing investigations of recent years strongly support the existence of marked sex differences in [olfactory] sensitivity in favour of women." Variations in olfactory sensitivity during the sexual cycle and during pregnancy, and deviation from normal in patients with endocrinological disorders, support the idea that sex hormones play an important role in determining the set point of olfactory acuity. However, the mechanisms underlying the hormonal influences have still to be clarified.

Hearing differences have also been well documented. The evidence is strong that females have greater threshold sensitivity than males to sound, especially for pure tones. This applies to all ages, with sex differences increasing with advancing age. Women show markedly lower tolerance to noise than men. Velle also cites the controversy surrounding the difference in lateralization of auditory output; however, from the data reviewed, men seem to be more lateralized than women for auditory verbal stimuli, whereas there are other indications that women are more lateralized for auditory, nonverbal stimuli.

There is general agreement that among adults, average visual acuity, both static and dynamic, is greater in men than in women. Velle also concludes from his reviews that men have better visual spatial ability than women. Also, marked sex differences have been reported in physiological responses to visual input.[2] Lateralization of visual stimuli appears to be more pronounced in men than in women. However, these are complex functions and therefore cannot be easily summarized. The literature is also voluminous, with some contradictory data. In other functions, such as processing verbal stimuli, women appear to perform better. These results may also reflect complex social behaviors as well as sensory differences.

## Infant Research

Early development is another interesting area of gender-difference research. There are response differences in male and female neonates, in both human and nonhuman primates. It is well established that newborns elicit responses in their caretakers and that caretaking is strongly affected by the temperament, responsiveness, state, and style of the infant. These responses have been studied by ethologists, psychologists, and more recently, psychoanalysts. Contrary to early ideas of the newborn as a "blank slate," or as "undifferentiated," neonates demonstrate a highly developed ability to elicit responses and to differentiate among many different stimuli. The relationship between newborns and their caretakers, usually mothers, is complex and mutually developed (Stern 1985). The interplay of innate characteristics and socialization contributes to the differences observed between males and females. Silverman, in a recent review (1987), suggests that the particular characteristics of female infants, including greater calmness and readiness to settle down, facilitate bonding with the mother. She further states, "parental behavior is elicited by a complex pattern of stimuli within the neonate—a pattern that signals and elicits accommodating responses from the mother" (p. 315). These studies emphasize the importance of early interactions between mother and child and suggest that these interactions "are the precursors of psychic structure."

This theory is consistent with the thinking of some psychoanalytic theorists such as Bowlby (1969), Fairbairn (1952), and Klein (1952), who emphasized the importance of the early relationships, and differs from Freud (1925), who did not place so much emphasis on the role of the preoedipal mother.

The particular importance in early development of the same-sex relationship (e.g., mother-daughter) has also received increasing attention. The earlier neurologic maturity and sensory responsiveness of the female have been thought to be factors facilitating the development of a different relationship between the mother and female infant than that between the mother and the male infant. Silverman summarizes much of this research from the 1970s and 1980s, writing that infant females demonstrate greater responsiveness in a number of sensory modalities. They show greater responsiveness to auditory signals (Friedman and Jacobs 1981; Lewis and Weinraub 1974; Osofsky and Conners 1979), sensitivity to tactile experiences (summarized in Korner 1974), and earlier face discrimination (Caron et al., 1982; Haviland and Malatesta 1981). The combination of greater sensory awareness and a more stable state system allows for beginning social exchanges between mother and daughter that a mother caring for the more fretful, less responsive male infant cannot attempt.

Obviously, the psychological issues, such as the identifications between a parent of the same sex as the infant and the child, are also likely to play an important role. "Gazing," the extended eye contact between mother and baby, is demonstrably important for all infants as a way of facilitating bonding between mother and her baby (Stern 1977, 1985). What is noteworthy in the current context, is the difference in the gazing of male and female infants apparent after the first day of birth. Female infants spend a greater percentage of time making eye contact than males. In addition, they make eye contact faster and, when involved in this activity, spend a longer period of time gazing than do males (summarized in Haviland and Malatesta 1981).

Vocalization, the forerunner of speech, does have an earlier start with females. Researchers report that female neonates vocalize more than males, and that parents vocalize more to daughters than to sons (Bell and Harper 1977; Brown 1979; Lewis and Weinraub 1974; Moss 1974). Rosenthal (1982) observed that mothers responded differentially to the gender of their offspring. Mothers vocalized when their daughters vocalized and when their sons moved. This difference may contribute to the proclivity for motor responses in males, which can lead to separation from mother, and vocalization in females, which enhances connectedness.

In sum, two different patterns emerge for girls and boys. Female neonates with their more stable state system, increased awareness of the outside world, and greater involvement in gazing and vocalization, show an increased potential for greater connectedness to the caregiver. Although bonding is clearly a task for all infants, small but important differences in male behavior may facilitate separation from the mother. The male's greater irritability and lessened responsiveness to calming and soothing make overstimulation a greater concern for the male neonate. The mother's animated face and her gazing, given the male's less stable state system, may be experienced as too arousing (Haviland and Malatesta 1981). An increase in fussiness, crying, or gaze aversion may follow from this overarousal.

All of these factors, together with the boy's preference for motor responses, lead to increased experience of separation. Although these generalizations do not account for the behavior of any one individual, they do suggest an early basis for what the infant brings to the early relationships that then shapes the future of those relationships.

This research suggests different patterns of interaction between caretakers and female and male infants. It suggests that girls' cognitive development and emotional life may also have a different configuration than boys', particularly concerning early bonding and the patterns of relationships.

The intricate blend of gender differences in responsiveness, differential parental encouragement of certain behaviors and responses according to culturally stereotyped concepts of male and female, and expectations of appropriate styles of each gender thus results in early gender role differences with important developmental implications. These differences may develop into stereotyped masculine and feminine styles. As more sophisticated data and concepts develop, the pathways of these relationships will become more clearly discernible.

## References

Bell RQ, Harper LV: Child Effects on Adults. Hillsdale, NJ, Lawrence Erlbaum, 1977

Bowlby J: Attachment and Loss, Vol 1: Attachment. New York, Basic Books, 1969

Brown CJ: Reactions of infants to their parents' voices. Infant Behavior and Child Development 2:295–300, 1979

Caron RF, Caron AJ, Myers RS: Abstraction of invariant face expression in infancy. Child Dev 53:1008–1015, 1982

Fairbairn WR: Psychoanalytic Studies of the Personality. London, Routledge & Kegan Paul, 1952

Freud S: Some psychical consequences of the anatomical distinction between the sexes (1925), in The Standard Edition of the Complete Psychological Works of Sigmund Freud, Vol 19. Translated and edited by Strachey J. London, Hogarth Press, 1961, pp 248–258

Freud S: Female sexuality (1931), in The Standard Edition of the Complete Psychological Works of Sigmund Freud, Vol 21. Translated and edited by Strachey J. London, Hogarth Press, 1961, pp 225–243

Friedman SL, Jacobs BL: Sex differences in neonatal behavior: responsiveness to repeated auditory stimulation. Infant Behavior and Development 4:175–183, 1981

Geschwind N, Levitsky I: Human brain: left-right asymmetries in temporal speech region. Science 161:186–187, 1968

Haviland JJ, Malatesta CZ: The development of sex differences in nonverbal signals: fallacies, facts and fantasies, in Gender and Nonverbal Behavior. Edited by Mayo G, Henley NM. New York, Springer-Verlag, 1981, pp 183–208

Henley N: Psychology and gender. Signs 11:101–119, 1985

Kandel E: Cellular mechanisms of learning and the biological basis of individuality, in Principles of Neural Science, 2nd Edition. Edited by Kandel E, Schwartz J. New York, Elsevier North-Holland, 1985, pp 816–833

Kelly D: Sexual differentiation of the nervous system, in Principles of Neural Science, 2nd Edition. Edited by Kandel E, Schwartz J. Elsevier North-Holland, 1985, pp 771–783

Klein M: Developments in Psychoanalysis. Edited by Riviere J. London, Hogarth Press, 1952

Korner AF: Methodological considerations in studying sex differences in the behavior functioning of newborns, in Sex Differences in Behavior. Edited by Friedman RC, Richart EM, Van de Wiele RL. New York, John Wiley, 1974

Kupferman I: Hemispheric asymmetrics and the cortical localization of higher cognitive and affective function, in Principles of Neural Science, 2nd Edition. Edited by Kandel E, Schwartz J. New York, Elsevier North-Holland, 1985, pp 673–687

Levy J: Perception of bilateral chimeric figures following hemispheric deconnection. Brain 95:61–78, 1972

Levy J: The origins of lateral asymmetry, in Lateralization in the Nervous System. Edited by Levy J. New York, Academic, 1977

Lewis M, Weinraub M: Sex of parent × sex of child: socioemotional development, in Sex Differences in Behavior. Edited by Friedman RC, Richart EM, Van de Wiele RL. New York, John Wiley, 1974, pp 165–190

Money J, Ehrhardt A: Man and Woman, Boy and Girl. Baltimore, MD, Johns Hopkins University Press, 1972

Moss HA: Early sex differentiation and mother-infant interaction, in Sex Differences in Behavior. Edited by Friedman RC, Richart EM, Van de Wiele RL. New York, John Wiley, 1974, pp 149–164

Osofsky J, Conners K: Mother-infant interaction: an interpretative view of a complex system, in Handbook of Infant Development. Edited by Osofsky J. New York, John Wiley, 1979, pp 519–549

Restak RM: The Brain: The Last Frontier. New York, Doubleday, 1979

Rosenthal MK: Vocal development in the neonatal period. Developmental Psychology 18:17–21, 1982

Silverman D: What are little girls made of? Psychoanalytic Psychology 4:315–334, 1987

Stern D: The First Relationship: Infant and Mother. Cambridge, MA, Harvard University Press, 1977

Stern D: The Interpersonal World of the Inpatient. New York, Basic Books, 1985

Velle W: Sex differences in sensory functions. Perspect Biol Med 30:490–522, 1987

Witelson S: Sex and the single hemisphere: right hemisphere specialization for spatial processing. Science 193:425–427, 1976

Witelson S: Les differences sexuelles dans la neurologie de la cognition: implications psychologiques, sociales, educatives et cliniques, in Le Fait Feminin. Edited by Sullerot E. Paris, France, Fayard, 1978, pp 287–303

Witelson S: The brain connection: the corpus callosum is larger in left-handers. Science 229:665–668, 1985a

Witelson S: An exchange on "gender." New York Review of Books, Oct 24, 1985b, pp 53–54

Witelson S: Research in neurology and cognitive psychology as to gender differences in brain functioning and related areas. Paper presented at the annual meeting of the American Psychiatric Association, Washington, DC, May 1986

## Editors' Notes

1. For another perspective, see Chapters 5 and 6 by Drs. Russo and Bleier, respectively.

2. See discussion in Chapters 5 and 6, by Drs. Russo and Bleier, respectively.

*Chapter 4*

# Sex Differences in the Brain: What They Are and How They Arise

## Bruce S. McEwen, Ph.D.

What is the basis of sex differences in behavior and brain function? Are sex differences acquired through learning or is a more innate substrate programmed by endocrine factors? In this chapter, I will briefly review the role of hormones in the development of the masculine and feminine neurological phenotypes. This phenotype is the substrate upon which learning and other environmental factors operate to develop the behavioral characteristics associated with the masculine and feminine personalities.

### Role of Sex Chromosomes and Sex Hormones

When considering biological sex differences, usually we first focus on the sex chromosomes. Indeed, in fetal life the sex chromosomes determine the sexual phenotype of the rest of the body, including the brain (Figure 1). The testes secrete testosterone during a critical period in early development when certain tissues are sensitive to this hormone (Huhtaniemi 1985); this testosterone secretion masculinizes and defeminizes various cellular structures throughout the brain and the reproductive organs. According to the present information, the female phenotype develops without specific hormonal influence because the ovaries are relatively quiescent during early development. Figure 2 presents a schematic view of androgen levels during devel-

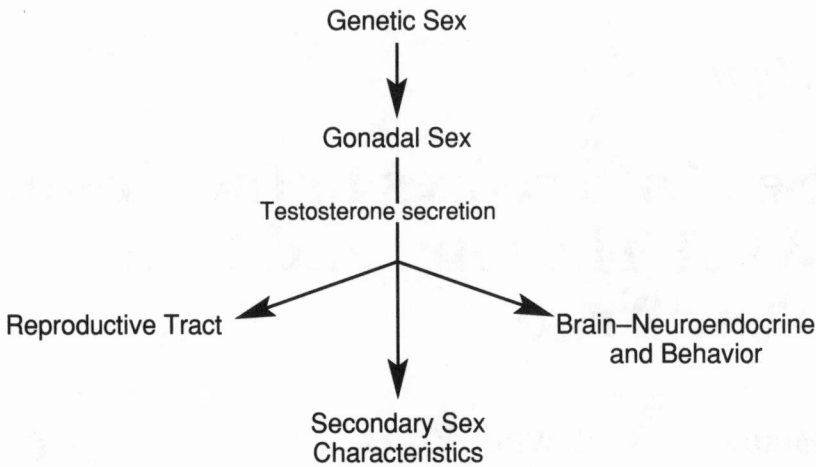

**Figure 1.** Brain and body sex are determined by secretion of testosterone during a sensitive period of early development. The sex of the gonad is determined by the genetic sex.

opment in the rat and in the human. In the human, an intermediate phase of androgen secretion lasts from birth through the first 2 years of neonatal life, but the significance of this phase is not yet established. The earliest phase of testosterone secretion in the human male fetus occurs between the 12th and 20th weeks of gestation (Abramovich and Rowe 1973); this phase is believed to masculinize the reproductive system and to initiate masculinization of the brain.

Masculinization, however, is a continuing process; later hormone actions and the individual's experiences both contribute to the further development of the sex differences. To begin to understand the nature of this process, we should consider some further details of the early phase of masculinization of the brain, as determined by experiments using the rat.

## Sexual Differentiation of the Rodent Brain

In the rat, we are aware of only two phases of androgen secretion, one perinatal and the other peripubertal and extending into adult life (Figure 2). It is the early phase that masculinizes the reproductive system and initiates masculinization of the brain. For this to occur, the brain must be sensitive enough to respond to the secreted andro-

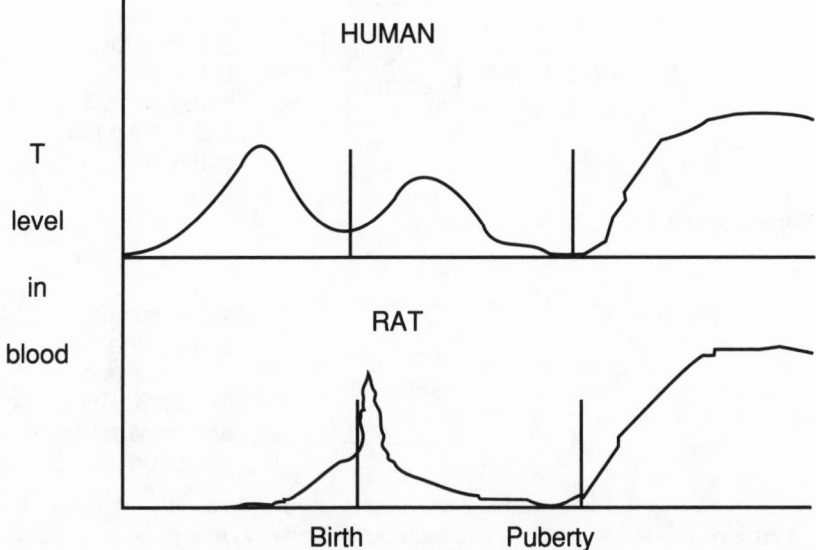

**Figure 2.** Testosterone (T) secretion patterns are shown in relation to developmental stages in human and rat. Redrawn from Huhtaniemi (1985).

gen. Receptor sites, which are specific protein molecules, bind the hormone and initiate a biological response (McEwen et al. 1982).

Receptors are produced by certain cells in the brain and in the anlage of the reproductive system and secondary sex tissues. The developmental actions of testosterone depend on two distinct receptor types, those that respond to androgens and those that respond to estrogens. This is because testosterone is converted by enzymes present in target tissues to form either a more active androgen, 5-alpha-dihydrotestosterone (5-alpha-DHT), or the potent estrogen estradiol (Figure 3). In the brain, both androgen and estrogen receptors, as well as the enzymes that convert testosterone to 5-alpha-DHT and to estradiol, are produced during the development that just precedes the first phase of testosterone secretion depicted in Figure 2. Of particular importance is the fact that males and females both produce the same complement of enzymes and receptors and hence are equally able to respond to testosterone, even though only the male secretes testosterone at the critical time in development. Thus, giving testosterone, or estradiol plus 5-alpha-DHT, to developing females will produce the same masculinization and defeminization that occurs naturally in the male (Goy and McEwen 1980; McEwen et al. 1982).

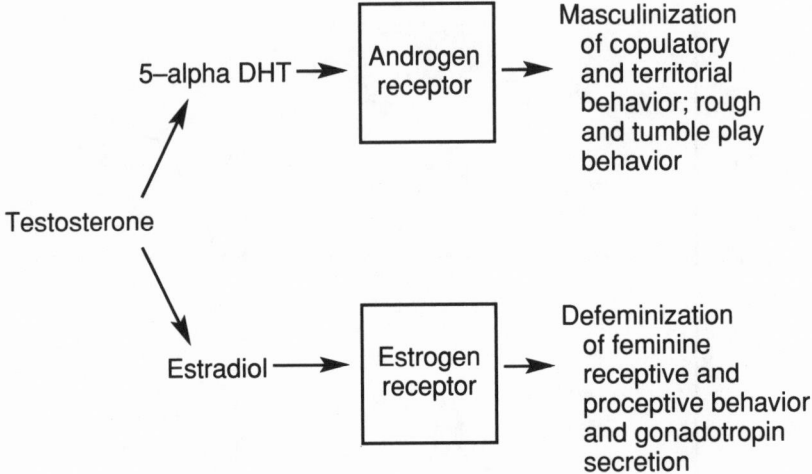

**Figure 3.** Testosterone produces its effects on brain sexual differentiation by being converted to more active metabolites by enzymes present in neural tissue; 5-alpha-dihydrotestosterone (5-alpha-DHT) and estradiol are the metabolites that bind to androgen and estrogen receptors, respectively, to produce effects indicated at right of figure.

## Masculinization and Defeminization

In describing sexual differentiation, I use the terms *masculinization* and *defeminization* to distinguish between two aspects of the process (Goy and McEwen 1980). *Defeminization* is the suppression of feminine characteristics that would otherwise develop in the absence of testosterone secretion, such as the ability to display feminine sexual behavior or cyclic ovulation. *Masculinization* is the enhancement of male characteristics that would otherwise not develop in the absence of testosterone secretion, such as masculine sexual and aggressive behavior. These two aspects of sexual differentiation are related to the two pathways of testosterone action: defeminization is linked to aromatization of testosterone (i.e., conversion of testosterone to estradiol) and to estrogen receptors, whereas masculinization is linked to DHT formation and to androgen receptors (Figure 3).

## Primary Events in Sexual Differentiation

The androgen and estrogen receptors mediate masculinization and defeminization in the cell nucleus of target cells. The cell nucleus contains the genetic information of the organism; it is a library of all the characteristics of all the cells of the body, which are organized into basic elements known as *genes*. Estrogen and androgen receptors act on certain genes through a specific molecular recognition mechanism and call forth the information within those genes, leading to the growth and functional differentiation of those cells. Sexual differentiation is thus a specific example of hormonally regulated development and differentiation of cell structure and function.

In the brain, the primary events associated with sexual differentiation are neuronal growth and increased functional specialization of groups of neurons (Arnold and Gorski 1984). Because the estrogen and androgen receptors appear in neurons after the final cell division has taken place, it is unlikely that testosterone has marked influences on neuronal proliferation (McEwen 1985). On the other hand, testosterone promotes growth of processes (called "neurites") from developing neurons, which are forming connections with other neurons (Toran-Allerand 1984). Because this growth occurs in neurons that have receptors and because the receptors are found only in certain nerve cells, the influence of testosterone on neural circuitry is very discrete and selective. Hence sex differences in brain circuitry, uncovered by the work of Raisman and Field (1973), are not large and are rather subtle. However, there is now a growing list of features of the nervous system that are different in males and females as a result of the early actions of testosterone.

Morphological differentiation of brain cells is linked to increased functional specialization; sexual differentiation promotes such specialization. One way this is manifested is in the actions of sex hormones in the adult brain. Adult brains of both sexes contain receptors for androgens and estrogens. Circulating androgens are found in females as well as in males; because of the conversion of testosterone to estradiol, which occurs in adult and developing brains, estrogen receptors play a functional role in the male brain as well as in the female brain. In other words, androgen and estrogen receptors are active in both sexes. Therefore, it is important that the effects of androgen and estrogen receptor activation in male and female brains are not exactly the same. The quantitative and qualitative sex differences in responses to estradiol, testosterone, and 5-alpha-DHT administration are indicative of functional sexual differentiation, possibly at the level of gene regulation (McEwen 1984).

One way these hormones affect functioning of the adult brain is by altering the amounts of neurochemicals that mediate transmission of electrical signals between anatomically connected nerve cells. This means that presence of circulating hormone changes the way that certain nerve cells communicate with each other and alters the way they respond to drugs. One of the consequences of the sexually different responses to estradiol, testosterone, and 5-alpha-DHT is that male and female brains do not necessarily respond to neurotransmitters and drugs in the same way. Actions of psychoactive drugs such as amphetamines, neuroleptics, and antidepressants are known to differ between men and women and, as a function of the hormonal status, to differ in premenopausal and postmenopausal women (Hamilton and Parry 1984). Hormones and sex differences thus play a noticeable role in psychopharmacology.

## Conclusions

What does all of this mean for our understanding of behavioral sex differences? It means that male and female brains begin postnatal life with subtle structural and functional differences that bias the input and output of information and modify the storage of experiences. Modern neuroscience teaches us that each experience and each psychological process involves neuronal activity and underlying chemical responses. The very chemistry of neurotransmission has the ability to modify nerve cell structure and function; these modifications can last for hours and may even lead to virtually permanent changes, as in learning. In fact, neurotransmitters, like hormones, can alter the expression of genes, leading to long-lasting changes in the brain.

The effect of hormones on genes is therefore only one facet of how nerve cell structure and function can change as a result of the environment. We should therefore be less concerned about the somewhat artificial distinction between "biological" factors such as hormones and "psychological" factors such as experiences because, in the final analysis, both sets of factors are able to influence brain cell structure and function and thus alter the substrate for behavior.

## References

Abramovich DR, Rowe P: Foetal plasma testosterone levels at mid-pregnancy and at term: relationship to foetal sex. J Endocrinol 55:621–622, 1973

Arnold AP, Gorski RA: Gonadal steroid induction of structural sex differences in the central nervous system. Annu Rev Neurosci 7:413–442, 1984

Goy RW, McEwen BS (eds): Sexual Differentiation of the Brain. Cambridge, MA, MIT Press, 1980

Hamilton J, Parry B: Sex-related differences in clinical drug response: implications for women's health. J Am Med Wom Assoc 38:126–132, 1984

Huhtaniemi I: Functional and regulatory differences between the fetal and adult populations of rat Leydig cells, in The Endocrine Physiology of Pregnancy and the Peripartal Period, Vol 21. Edited by Jaffe R, Dell'Acqua S. New York, Raven, 1985, pp 64–85

McEwen BS: Gonadal hormone receptors in developing and adult brain: relationship to the regulatory phenotype, in Fetal Neuroendocrinology. Edited by Elledorff F, Gluckman P, Parvizi N. Ithaca, NY, Perinatology Press, 1984, pp 149–159

McEwen BS: Steroid hormone receptors and actions in the developing brain, in The Endocrine Physiology of Pregnancy and the Peripartal Period, Vol 21. Edited by Jaffe R, Dell'Acqua S. New York, Raven, 1985, pp 183–193

McEwen BS, Biegon A, Davis P, et al: Steroid hormones: humoral signals which alter brain cell properties and functions. Recent Prog Horm Res 38:41–92, 1982

Raisman G, Field P: Sexual dimorphism in the neutrophil of the preoptic area of the rat and its dependence on neonatal androgen. Brain Res 54:1–29, 1973

Toran-Allerand CD: On the genesis of sexual differentiation of the central nervous system: morphogenetic consequences of steroidal exposure and possible role of alphafetoprotein. Prog Brain Res 61:63–98, 1984

## Chapter 5

# Reconstructing the Psychology of Women: An Overview

## Nancy Felipe Russo, Ph.D.

In challenging traditional paradigms, feminist scholars have argued for research that connects social, economic, and political contexts to psychological dynamics (Carmen et al. 1981; Fine 1985; Sherif 1979; Sonderegger 1985; Walker 1984). The new scholarship on the psychology of women (Caplan 1985a, 1985b; Deaux 1985; Howell and Bayes 1981; Rieker and Carmen 1984) has forced formal professional institutions and individual researchers to examine psychology's theories and methods.

In this chapter, I will discuss these efforts to eliminate sex bias in research, identifying special implications for mental health researchers, particularly regarding the mental health effects of women's changing roles at work and in the family.

Although the recommendations developed by the various disciplines overlap, they are not identical. While I have drawn on all of them in developing this discussion, I rely most heavily on the work of the Committee on the Status of Women of the American Sociological Association (1980), the Task Force on Nonsexist Research of the Division of the Psychology of Women of the American Psychological Association (1983), and the discussions of the ad hoc Committee on Nonsexist Research of the American Psychological Association which I have participated in over the last 4 years. I would also like to thank D. Allen Meyer for his comments on the manuscript and Ria Hermann and Rebecca Huey for their help in assembling reference materials.

## Sex Bias in Research

Efforts to eliminate sex bias in research have a twofold impact. First, these efforts expand the knowledge based on women's experiences. Neglected areas such as the menstrual cycle, contraception and abortion, lesbian issues, women's friendships, rape, and wife battering are now considered legitimate and important research topics. Second, and perhaps more important, such efforts force shifts in basic concepts and accepted ways of conducting the scientific enterprise, raising questions about the quality of research.

Sex-biased assumptions are found in all stages of the research process: how questions are asked; the ways variables are conceptualized, measured, and labeled; the design and analysis of results; and the interpretation of findings. Psychological theories have not had equal relevance to both genders, and greater value and attention have been given to the culture and experience of males. "Man" has surely been the measure of all things psychological.

### The Importance of Asking the Right Questions

Increasing the number of women in science, it has been argued, will change science. This assertion stems from asking how scientific questions are generated. Courses in research methods teach students that questions are derived from theory and previous research. More likely, however, the researcher asks, "Why did that happen to me (or to a relative or acquaintance)?" and then begins the literature search for a theory and relevant research. As long as men and women have different experiences and are subject to different sex role expectations, they will be likely to generate different hypotheses and hold different areas of concern.

White, middle-class males continue to be disproportionately overrepresented as researchers, particularly in institutions with adequate research resources (Russo 1985). Thus analytical frameworks and models that are generated from the experiences of the researcher are limited, as are the research questions asked and the interpretations offered. The most critical area for future efforts is asking the right questions.

Although gender is a significant variable in the development, diagnosis, and treatment of mental disorders, it is not often conceptualized into theories to explain mental disorder. Gender differences in the rates and patterns of diagnoses are so dramatic that a basic test of any theory purporting to explain the etiology of mental disorder must be the ability to account for those differences (Russo 1985).

Research questions are framed so that they implicitly or explicitly apply to only one sex. For example, questions are asked about the mental health impact of mothers' employment on children, but not that of fathers. Job-related characteristics are assumed to affect men's adaptation to work, factors at home to determine women's adjustment. When individuals of either sex, but particularly women, behave in ways that are inconsistent with gender and sex role stereotypes, they are seen as exhibiting pathology.

Psychological theories have incorporated male sex role expectations as ideals of maturity and adjustment. Male-oriented developmental tasks of autonomy and separation have been valued over the connectedness and responsibility for others that characterize women's roles (Gilligan 1982). Research on these characteristics of connectedness and responsibility would provide some understanding of the link between women's psychological characteristics and their social roles and would provide a sophisticated advance over earlier approaches. Achieving such advances, however, requires avoiding the traditional error of attributing women's judgments and behaviors entirely to personality traits rather than to their interaction with an environment that enforces female sex role obligations and male power and privilege.

### The Pervasiveness and Subtlety of Sex Bias

Unexamined assumptions about the sexes affect the research process at all stages, and methodologically flawed studies supporting gender stereotypes are widely cited without mention of their limitations. Primary sources need to be reviewed, particularly for sexist assumptions and unwarranted generalizations. McHugh et al. (1986) have pointed out that excessive confidence in and reliance on traditional methods of research contribute to sex bias and point to the need to question how questions are asked and how data are gathered.

Analyses of sex bias in research are becoming increasingly sophisticated. They have progressed from identifying the obvious—for example, women not being included in a study purporting to describe human behavior—to the subtle—for example, changes in beta weight outcomes depending on the order that variables are forced into a regression equation. The subtleties reveal inadequacies in theoretical models as well as methods (Grady 1981; Sherif 1979, 1982).

*Sample Selection.* Sample selection issues in mental health research are all too often ignored. A basic flaw has been the use of male participants in research that is then generalized to all humans. The use of single-sex samples can result in a skewed knowledge base. In the case of clinical drug testing, which by the mandate of the Food and Drug Administration excludes women from early trials, such incomplete data can be potentially life threatening if harmful side effects that occur only in women are not detected (Hamilton et al. 1984).

Samples may be haphazard or not adequately controlled for life span stage. For example, one might ask whether research on differences between parenting styles of fathers and mothers reflects only gender differences or also relative ages of fathers and mothers.

Gender representativeness of a sample should be considered. In particular, clinical samples should not be used to make statements about all women. The extent to which institutions or settings filter males and females differently may affect the research findings. For example, many sex and race differences found in studies of patients in state and county mental hospitals are not found in studies of patients in private mental hospitals (Russo and Sobel 1981).

In designing research and specifying the sample, insufficient attention is given to variables that correlate with group membership. In drug research, weight, body composition, and total body water differ by sex and are known to affect drug responsivity, yet drug dosages are often fixed or controlled only for weight (Hamilton et al. 1984).

***Situational Characteristics.***    Situations may differ in their salience, familiarity, relevance, and meaning for males and females (Task Force on Nonsexist Research 1983). Sex-by-situation interactions are found more frequently than main effects for sex (Deaux 1976). This may hold for the diagnostic context as well (Russo and Sobel 1981). Sex-related differences in a behavior (e.g., conformity) may reflect a greater use of male-related research tasks (Sistrunk and McDavid 1971). Selection of such tasks may reflect subtle experimenter bias about what is appropriate for males and females. For example, Frodi et al. (1977) observed that studies of aggression using male participants were more likely to use behavioral measures, while those using females were more likely to use paper and pencil tests of aggression.

Sex of experimenter, sex composition of the group, and presence of others affect problem-solving performance in females in particular (Dweck and Bush 1976; Eagly 1978, 1983; Harris 1971; Ruble and Higgins 1976; Taylor and Fiske 1978). For example, females have been reported to perform less well on a variety of tasks when in the presence of males. In mixed-sex groups, females show poorer levels of achievement than in single-sex groups, although stressing the importance of effort to success in the task instructions can improve their performance (LaNoue and Curtis 1985). More research is needed on the aspects of the research situation that result in sex-related differences with implications for mental health.

***Questionnaire and Instrument Development.*** Psychological research, testing, and evaluation instruments should be reviewed to ensure that no offensive and inappropriate language or questions are included; that material relevant to women and minorities is included; that validity evidence for women and minorities is available where relevant; and that factors unrelated to the construct being measured do not interfere with group performance (American Educational Research Association 1985).

In performance measures, particularly regarding research on abilities, length of time before responding may reflect many psychological variables, including motivation and test anxiety as well as willingness to take risks and to sacrifice accuracy for speed. For example, low anxious boys perform best under time pressure conditions compared with other groups of children, and their performance is enhanced by evaluative pressure; anxious girls will strive for accuracy at the cost of speed under time pressure (Hill 1984; Plass and Hill 1986). Thus, research that purports to discover sex-related differences in abilities must be carefully conducted and evaluated so that gender differences in performance do not become inappropriately attributed to biological differences between the sexes.

Although test publishers have recognized the existence of racial bias in tests developed by white, middle-class researchers and standardized on white, middle-class students, only recently have the effects of sex bias on test development been examined (Campbell 1981). The wording of questions is biased, tests are not validated on representative groups, and insufficient care is given to the characteristics of the experimental setting that can result in gender differences in responses. Questions should be phrased to allow for the full range of possible answers. For example, the question, "Do you believe that female psychiatrists are as intelligent as male psychiatrists?" does not allow for the possibility that female psychiatrists are more intelligent than their male colleagues.

In ability tests, early research documented the effects of bias in content of test problems, with boys doing better on test problems dealing with stereotypically masculine activities (Coffman 1961; Milton 1957). Adolescent girls are more likely to get an item correct on an achievement test if it mentions more girls than boys or equal numbers of girls (Donlon et al. 1971).

Even the format of a test can create gender differences in performance. For a wide range of subjects, including mathematics and reading comprehension, switching from essay or fill-in-the-blank questions to objective items such as multiple choice produces higher scores for males (Dwyer 1979; Murphy 1977).

Widely used research instruments, such as life event scales, require substantial revision. For example, life event inventories do not include stressful events common in women's lives, such as abortion and rape, yet they do include events that are less likely to be experienced by women, such as entering or leaving the armed forces. Such inventories fail to incorporate indicators of personal and situational resource deficits, and are thus insensitive to the effects of enduring conditions that are more likely to affect women, such as problems in intimate relationships, poverty, or poor health (Newmann 1986).

Diagnostic instruments used in research are also deficient. For example, the masculinity-femininity scale of the Minnesota Multiphasic Personality Inventory has been widely used in research despite shaky scientific underpinnings. Validation of that scale originally consisted of identifying items that discriminated between a group of 117 male armed services personnel versus a group of 108 female workers and 17 male homosexuals (Campbell 1981).

The assumption persists that male and female behavior is bipolar, on a unidimensional continuum, but there are differences in interpretations of the meaning of concepts. As Kaplan (1983) has pointed out, men who rely on others to cook, clean, and find their socks are not labeled "dependent." Men's inability to express themselves has not been called an "emotional defect." The willingness to endure pain and risk bodily injury for financial security has not been labeled "masochism" if the behavior involved is boxing or football. The debate on how to conceptualize masculinity and femininity continues (Spence 1985).

Instruments used to measure depression have not always separated the presence of dysphoric mood, or "sadness," from other depressive symptoms, including loss of interest in normal activities, self-reproach, feelings of worthlessness, and suicidal thoughts or behaviors (Klerman 1980). The sex-related difference in composite depression scores appears to reflect the greater levels of sadness reported by women (Newmann 1984).

### Nonsexist Language

Language shapes our thinking, and nonsexist language is essential for nonsexist research (Martyna 1980; Moulton et al. 1978). Nonsexist language is considered so basic that the American Psychological Association has incorporated nonsexist language guidelines in its widely used *Publication Manual* (1983). Those guidelines point to the importance of precise language: generic and sex-specific terms should be used appropriately, and parallel terms for males and females should be used in parallel situations. For example, in describing households headed by mothers, it is misleading to refer to them as "single-parent families"; wife abuse is the significant social problem, not "spouse" abuse; one should not refer to "men and girls" if adults of both sexes are being discussed; men should not be addressed as "Dr." and women as "Ms." if both are physicians.

Another problem is the tendency for negative labels to become attached to the nontraditional. Nontraditional behaviors are considered maladaptive, particularly if they are associated with opposite gender, although there may be no research support of that assumption. Thus, when boys play with dolls they are labeled as having "gender identity confusion," and career dedication by women is considered "masculine." Nontraditional behavior leads to other types of negative value judgments. For example, providing for the economic welfare of the family is evidence of being a "good" father, but not a "good" mother (McHugh et al. 1986).

A number of studies show that language can subtly reinforce stereotypes. In an uncritical and misleading yet widely cited summary of sex difference research, Garai and Scheinfeld (1968) found that females scored higher on 41 comparisons and males on 35 comparisons. Parlee (1975) pointed out, however, that use of certain descriptors in their article led to the impression that males' performance was "better" than that of females. When females scored higher than males, their performance was described as "superior" only 27% of the time.

Labeling transforms statistical differences into innate differences. Traits found in both sexes—for example, aggression, nurturance, dependency—become labeled as either "masculine" or "feminine." Individuals who exhibit a trait labeled as belonging to the other sex become defined as deviant, pathological, or exceptional and may be demeaned for violation of sex role norms.

### Observer Bias

Observers rate individuals differently based on gender and sex role stereotypes, even where products and performances of men and women are identical (Geis et al. 1982). Violations of sex role norms in particular result in biased observer judgments. Sex-related differences based on observational data, particularly clinical observations, should be substantiated through other data collection methods (American Educational Research Association 1985).

Coie et al. (1974) found that persons acting in a manner incongruent with their sex role were viewed as more maladjusted than individuals acting in a sex-role-congruent manner. Costrich et al. (1975) found that an aggressive woman was rated as even more dominant than an aggressive man with identical scripts. The consequences for sex role deviance appear to be more severe for females compared with males in some contexts (Feinman 1981; O'Leary et al. 1980; Shaffer and Johnson 1980).

Rosenfeld (1982) examined the relationship between stereotype violation and treatment decisions in a psychiatric emergency room. For disorders in which females predominate (neuroses and depression), males were significantly more likely to be hospitalized than females. For disorders in which males predominate (personality disorders and substance abuse), females were more likely than males to be hospitalized. The study focused on a limited population and did not explore the interaction of patient characteristics such as race/ethnicity, marital and parental status, education, and employment with the decision to hospitalize. However, the findings do suggest an important relationship between sex role violation and diagnostic judgments (this may also reflect pathology).

### Interpretation and Conclusions

Researchers' willingness to generate conclusions based more on stereotypes than on data continues to be a significant problem. In interpreting research results, conclusions that support discrimination and devaluation of women are often improperly drawn. For example, the assumption that spatial ability underlies achievement in science and mathematics is not supported by empirical research (Linn and Petersen 1983; Meece et al. 1982). Sex-related differences in spatial ability emerge prior to adolescence and are related to specific types of skills, such as mental rotation of figures and tests of horizontality and verticality. No differences have been documented in tasks requiring an analytic, sequential strategy, which is closer to those skills required in scientific reasoning (Linn and Petersen 1983), yet research on gender differences in spatial ability is still used to "explain" why women have not achieved as much success in science as men.

Researchers should closely relate their conclusions to their results and should consider the size as well as the statistical significance of any gender differences. A common error in analyzing sex-related differences is concluding that sex differences exist without application of appropriate statistical tests. If a correlation coefficient involving one sex but not the other is statistically significant, a sex difference cannot be said to exist without statistically testing the difference between the correlations (Sherman 1978).

Selective reporting of results can also affect conclusions. For example, if the income of black women is compared with that of white women rather than that of black men, one can conclude that black women are advantaged over black men because the income differential between black women and white women is smaller than that between black men and white men. A different conclusion is drawn when one also considers that black men earn 1.5 times the salary of black women (Campbell 1981).

In reporting results to the public, mental health professionals have an ethical and social responsibility to recognize the potential for misinterpretation and take steps to avoid it. This is true for all research. For example, in October 1984, the morning news carried the assertion that, contrary to earlier research, "new" research had established that there were no sex differences in mental disorders. Press conference materials distributed in conjunction with publication of the preliminary results from the National Institute of Mental Health's Epidemiologic Catchment Area Study (Myers et al. 1984; Robins et al. 1984) contained statements asserting that the study's failure to find gender differences in total overall rates of the disorders covered was a new and significant contribution and contradicted earlier work. In fact, the findings confirmed the thrust of earlier work, which had pointed to extensive sex-related differences in rates of specific mental disorders. Further, the overall rate of mental disorder referred to in the preliminary findings reflected the rates of only the particular 15 disorders chosen for inclusion in the study. The subsequent widespread publicity hampered efforts to draw attention to the continued importance of understanding the effects of gender and sex roles in the development, diagnosis, and treatment of mental disorders because time and energy had to be spent refuting the erroneous interpretations. For researchers to assert that their work was misinterpreted is not sufficient. Even if the interpretations are incorrect, the results of research have been used to support the status quo. When reporting findings, special care must be taken to minimize the opportunity for inappropriate interpretations.

## Reconstructing a Picture of Women's Lives That Mirrors Their Realities

Feminists are going beyond critiquing sex bias in theories and methods and are reconstructing the knowledge base about women's experiences to include an understanding of women's changing roles and circumstances. Major changes include the dramatic increase in labor force participation of women, particularly women with young children. Women have also gained increased control over childbearing, and life expectancy for women has increased significantly compared with that for men. At the same time, occupational segregation is still pervasive. Further, there are more households headed by women, and more women live in poverty (Russo and Denmark 1984).

Some of the recent findings related to the effects of women's work and family roles on mental health are summarized here as a step toward constructing the complex picture of women's changing realities.

### Marriage, Employment, and Mental Health

Marital status is a powerful predictor of mental health. The relationship between marital status and home life satisfaction is much stronger for men than women; married men appear to be in better mental health than married women (Gove et al. 1983). In contrast, the relationship between the quality of marriage and home life satisfaction is much stronger for married women than for married men. This difference may reflect different psychological functions of marriage for husband and wife. Men gain more instrumentally from marriage than women do. That is, men receive housekeeping and other services, while women appear to invest more emotionally in marriage than do men (Gove et al. 1983). The positive relationship between marriage and mental health appears to reflect more than companionship or a satisfying sex life.

The effects of women's employment on mental health appear to depend on their marital, parental, and economic status. Married women play multiple roles, and the combination of working and having children appears to contribute to depressive symptomatology for women, but not for men (Cleary and Mechanic 1983). However, economic factors interact with sex roles. For working-class mothers with young children, paid employment appears to create a benefit because it raises the level of stress from life events that can be tolerated before one develops psychiatric symptomatology (Parry 1986).

Compared with housewives, employed married women with lower incomes appear to be more affected by stress caused by child rearing, but less affected by other life events. It may be that employment creates difficulties in caring for children, but provides a buffer for other types of stress experienced by lower-income women. Because this relationship is not found for women with higher incomes, the time and work demands for women who cannot afford to purchase assistance may underlie the relationship of child rearing, employment, and depression (Cleary and Mechanic 1983). Psychosocial studies of how time and work demands are actually handled by those lower-income women who avoid depression would be extremely helpful in developing prevention strategies.

Few developmental studies extend over the entire life-cycle. Variables that may relate to employment and well-being vary with life stage. A recent study of employed married rural women with children of high school age reported that the only family-related variable related to job satisfaction was children's support for their mother's working. The other major predictors of women's satisfaction with the multiple roles of worker and mother were job related, including job performance progress, duties, and reason for working (McHenry et al. 1985).

Mental health indicators have converged for the sexes; the association of employment with improved psychological well-being and mental health for women has been identified as a major source of this convergence (Kessler and McRae 1981, 1983; McLanahan and Glass 1985). Another reason offered is the possible negative impact of wives' employment on the mental health of their husbands. However, other factors affecting men's mental health are also correlated with the work force participation of wives. For example, a closer look at mental health indicators for men reveals that their distress levels are directly related to their earnings (Kessler 1979, 1982). Wives' employment is also negatively correlated with husbands' job satisfaction, suggesting that the reported association between wives' employment and husbands' mental health may also reflect the quality of the husband's work environment (Staines et al. 1985).

Economic hardship—associated with low income, low education, youth, and having young children—is related to depression in both sexes, and wives' employment is related to economic hardship. Ross and Huber (1985), who studied a national sample of married couples, found an inverse relationship between a husband's personal earnings and depression (the more the earnings, the less the likelihood of depression). No such relationship was found for wives.

The impact of wives' employment on husbands' distress and marital satisfaction depends on the personality characteristics and attitudes of the working couple. Ross et al. (1983) reported that the relationship between husbands' distress and wives' employment was found in couples where the preference of both husband and wife was for the wife to stay at home. Research on dual-worker married couples with preschool children reported that individuals with high levels of

both instrumental and expressive personality characteristics (androg-
ynous persons) experienced the highest levels of marital satisfaction
(Chassin et al. 1985). In addition, couples who had similar attitudes
toward women's roles had higher levels of marital satisfaction. Perceived control over the choice to work is also related to marital satisfaction in dual-career couples (Alvarez 1985). Thus, unless such
variables as the economic status of the family and the attitudes of
both spouses are examined, conclusions about reasons for the convergence of mental health indicators for the sexes can be misleading.
Married men still do better than married women on mental health
indicators. Men in the labor force show lower levels of psychological
distress than women in the labor force, and homemakers exhibit
higher levels than both groups (Kessler and McLeod 1984). If the level
of economic hardship is controlled, the presence of children is associated with decreased levels of depression.

Increases in women's education have contributed to increases in
women's mental well-being. Education is a significant preventive
against depression, perhaps because it may lead to a greater sense of
mastery and control, which are necessary conditions for the development of active problem-solving approaches. Kessler (1982) and
Kessler and McRae (1982) reported that whether or not women were
employed, education is more important than earnings or family income in predicting distress. For wives, lower educational levels and
the presence of young children are associated with more depression
(Kessler 1982). Employment outside the home does not appear to
protect a woman from depression independent of education (Warren
and McEachren 1985).

Evidence suggests that professional women are less likely than
nonprofessional women to exhibit depressive symptoms, perhaps because of their higher education (Warren and McEachren 1985). Employment, professional or nonprofessional, outside the home is also
related to a more autonomous sense of self, while derived identity is
related to higher levels of depressive symptomatology (Warren and
McEachren 1983).

### Sources of Stress in Women's Lives

Evidence suggests that women experience stressful life events more
often than do men (Aneshensel et al. 1981; Cleary and Mechanic 1983;
Gore and Mangione 1983). They are more likely to experience the
absence of a spouse, social isolation, economic hardship, and chronic
health problems (Newmann 1986). Women report significantly more
exposure to death than do men (Kessler and McLeod 1984) and are

also more likely to experience rape and other forms of violence (Koss 1990). Women appear to have greater vulnerability than men to stress arising from interpersonal problems (Kessler and McLeod 1984; Newmann 1984), while men are more vulnerable to stress related to their provider role such as job stress or income loss (Kessler and McLeod 1984; Radloff and Rae 1981).

Research on coping strategies in different situations is needed. Some research suggests that women selectively ignore stresses related to work and finances. However, when they are married and mothers, women combine the more active strategy of seeking advice with other forms of passive coping, for example, resignation and passive acceptance (Fleishman 1984). Recent research on which life events engender stress in men and women suggests that the greater involvement of women in the lives of others is a major contributor to the association between gender and emotional distress. When men and women were asked to identify events considered distressing, women reported distress in response to life crises occurring in members of their family, friends, and neighbors, while men seldom mentioned such events. Although men do appear as distressed as women by life crises affecting their spouses and children, they do not show concern in the same way that women do for individuals beyond the immediate family unit (Kessler and McLeod 1984).

More research is needed on how female sex role obligations create women's greater responsivity to stress. The mental health implications of being asked to perform helping roles have not been explored, despite some data indicating that social networks can be so demanding that women are in better mental health if they are isolated from other members of the network (Cohler and Lieberman 1980).

The interactive effects of gender and ethnicity on mental health have been documented in research on the use of mental health facilities (Russo and Olmedo 1983; Russo and Sobel 1981). Race and socioeconomic factors also interact so that racial differences in psychological distress are enhanced among people with low incomes, particularly poor black women (Kessler and Neighbors 1986). As Kessler and Neighbors have pointed out (p. 113), we must "go beyond social class to search for determinants of race differences in distress." To do this appropriately requires simultaneously examining gender effects.

## Looking to the Future

Recently feminist scholarship has challenged old paradigms and, in that challenge, has revitalized the mental health professions. Feminists have begun to define women's experiences in their own terms. These new constructions will create new conceptions of the human experience of both women and men. Recognizing the diversity of women is critical. Problems of minority women, disabled women, young women, and elderly women differ. However, all women are affected by sex role stereotyping and discrimination.

Although men and women are more similar than different, it is clear that men and women behave differently. We have yet to understand adequately the processes that create these differences. Research on the psychology of women that provides knowledge about women's lives and suggests positive strategies for change in their roles and status will create a foundation for the primary prevention of mental disorders.

# References

Alvarez W: The meaning of maternal employment for mothers and their perceptions of their three year old children. Child Dev 56:360–380, 1985

American Educational Research Association: AERA guidelines for eliminating race and sex bias in educational research and evaluation. Educational Researcher 14:16–17, 1985

American Psychological Association: Publication Manual of the American Psychological Association, 3rd Edition. Washington, DC, American Psychological Association, 1983

Aneshensel C, Frerichs R, Clark V: Family roles and sex differences in depression. J Health Soc Behav 22:379–393, 1981

Campbell PB: The impact of societal biases on research methods. National Institute of Education, U.S. Department of Education, 1981

Caplan PJ (ed): Feminist psychology: single life and married life, women's sexuality. International Journal of Women's Studies—Special Issue 8(1): whole issue, 1985a

Caplan PJ (ed): Feminist psychology: women in groups, sex roles and sex differences. International Journal of Women's Studies—Special Issue 8(4): whole issue, 1985b

Carmen EH, Russo N, Miller J: Inequality and women's mental health: an overview. Am J Psychiatry 138:1319–1330, 1981

Chassin L, Cooper K, Zeiss A: Self-role congruence and marital satisfaction in dual worker couples with preschool children. Social Psychology 48:301–312, 1985

Cleary PD, Mechanic D: Sex differences in psychological distress among married people. J Health Soc Behav 24:111–121, 1983

Coffman WE: Sex differences in response to items in an achievement test, in The Yearbook of the National Council on Measurement in Education, 18th Edition. Ames, IA, National Council on Measurement in Education, 1961, pp 117–124

Cohler B, Lieberman M: Social relations and mental health among three European ethnic groups. Res Aging 2:445–469, 1980

Coie JD, Pennington BR, Buckley HH: Effects of situational stress and roles on the attribution of psychological disorder. J Clin Consult Psychol 42:559–568, 1974

Committee on the Status of Women in Sociology: Sexist biases in sociological research: problems and issues. ASA Footnotes 1:8–9, 1980

Costrich N, Feinstein J, Kiddler L, et al: When stereotypes hurt: studies of penalties for role reversals. J Exp Soc Psychol 11:520–530, 1975

Deaux K: The Behavior of Women and Men. Monterey, CA, Brooks/Cole, 1976

Deaux K: Sex and gender. Ann Rev Psychol 36:49–81, 1985

Donlon TF, Ekstrom RB, Lockheed ME: The consequences of sex bias in the content of major achievement test batteries. Measurement and Evaluation in Guidance 11:202–216, 1971

Dweck CS, Bush E: Sex differences in learned helplessness, I: differential debilitation with peer and adult evaluations. Developmental Psychology 12:147–156, 1976

Dwyer CA: The role of tests and their construction in producing apparent sex-related differences, in Sex-Related Differences in Cognitive Functioning. Edited by Wittig MA, Petersen AC. New York, Academic, 1979, pp 335–353

Eagly AH: Sex differences in influenceability. Psychol Bull 85:86–116, 1978

Eagly AH: Gender and social influence: a social psychological analysis. Am Psychol 38:971–982, 1983

Feinman S: Why is cross-sex-role behavior more approved for girls than for boys? a status characteristics approach. Sex Roles 7:289–300, 1981

Fine M: Reflections on a feminist psychology of women: paradoxes and prospects. Psychology of Women Quarterly 9:167–183, 1985

Fleishman JA: Personality characteristics and coping patterns. J Health Soc Behav 25:229–244, 1984

Frodi A, Macaulay J, Thome PR: Are women always less aggressive than men? a review of the experimental literature. Psychol Bull 84:634–660, 1977

Garai JE, Scheinfeld A: Sex differences in mental and behavioral traits. Genet Psychol Monogr 77:169–299, 1968

Geis FL, Carter MR, Butler DJ: Research on Seeing and Evaluating People. Newark, University of Delaware, 1982

Gilligan C: In a Different Voice: Psychological Theory and Women's Development. Cambridge, MA, Harvard University Press, 1982

Gore S, Mangione TW: Social roles, sex roles, and psychological distress: relative and interactive models of sex differences. J Health Soc Behav 24:300–312, 1983

Gove WR, Hughes M, Style C: Does marriage have positive effects on psychological well-being of the individual? J Health Soc Behav 24:122–131, 1983

Grady KE: Sex bias in research design. Psychology of Women Quarterly 5:628–636, 1981

Hamilton JA, Lloyd C, Alagna SW, et al: Gender, depressive subtypes, and gender-age effects on anti-depressant response: hormonal hypotheses. Psychopharmacol Bull 23:475–480, 1984

Harris S: Influence of subject and experimenter sex in psychological research. J Consult Clin Psychol 37:291–294, 1971

Hill KT: Debilitating motivation and testing: a major educational problem, possible solutions, and policy applications, in Research on Motivation in Education: Student Motivation, Vol 1. Edited by Ames R, Ames C. New York, Academic, 1984, pp 245–274

Howell E, Bayes M (eds): Women and Mental Health. New York, Basic Books, 1981

Kaplan M: A woman's view of DSM-III. Am Psychol 38:786–792, 1983

Kessler RC: Stress, social status, and psychological distress. J Health Soc Behav 20:259–272, 1979

Kessler RC: A disaggregation of the relationship between socioeconomic status and psychological distress. Am Sociol Rev 47:752–764, 1982

Kessler RC, McLeod JD: Sex differences in vulnerability to undesirable life events. Am Sociol Rev 49:620–631, 1984

Kessler RC, McRae JA: Trends in sex and psychological distress. Am Sociol Rev 46:443–452, 1981

Kessler RC, McRae JA: The effect of wives' employment on the mental health of married men and women. Am Sociol Rev 47:217–227, 1982

Kessler RC, McRae JA: Trends in the relationship between sex and attempted suicide. J Health Soc Behav 24:98–110, 1983

Kessler RC, Neighbors HW: A new perspective on the relationships among race, social class, and psychological distress. J Health Soc Behav 27:107–115, 1986

Klerman GL: Overview of affective disorders, in Comprehensive Textbook of Psychiatry III, Vol 2. Edited by Kaplan HI, Freedman AM, Sadock BI. Baltimore, MD, Williams & Wilkins, 1980, pp 1305–1319

Koss MP: The Women's Mental Health Research Agenda: Violence against women. Am Psychol 45:374–380, 1990

LaNoue JB, Curtis RC: Improving women's performance in mixed-sex situations by effort attributions. Psychology of Women Quarterly 9:337–356, 1985

Linn MC, Petersen AC: Emergence and characterization of gender differences in spatial ability: a meta-analysis. Unpublished manuscript, University of California, Berkeley, 1983

Martyna W: Beyond the "he/man" approach: the case for non-sexist language. Signs 5:482–493, 1980

McHenry PC, Hamdorf KG, Walters CM, et al: Family and job influences onrole satisfaction of employed rural mothers. Psychology of Women Quarterly 9:242–257, 1985

McHugh MC, Koeske RD, Frieze IH: Issues to consider in conducting nonsexist psychological research: a guide for researchers. Am Psychol 41:879–890, 1986

McLanahan SS, Glass JL: A note on the trend in sex differences in psychological distress. J Health Soc Behav 26:328–335, 1985

Meece JL, Eccles-Parsons, Kaczala CM, et al: Sex differences in math achievement: toward a model of academic choice. Psychol Bull 91:324–348, 1982

Milton GA: The effects of sex role identification upon problem solving skills. J Abnorm Soc Psychol 55:208–212, 1957

Moulton J, Robinson GM, Elias C: Sex bias in language use: neutral pronouns that aren't. Am Psychol 33:1032–1036, 1978

Murphy RC: Sex differences in examination performance. Paper presented to the International Conference on Sex Role Stereotyping, Cardiff, Wales, 1977

Myers JK, Weissman MM, Tischler GL, et al: Six-month prevalence of psychiatric disorders in three communities. Arch Gen Psychiatry 41:959–967, 1984

Newmann JP: Sex differences in symptoms of depression: clinical disorder or normal distress? J Health Soc Behav 25:136–159, 1984

Newmann JP: Gender, life strains, and depression. J Health Soc Behav 27:161–178, 1986

O'Leary VE, Kahn A, Wever-Kollman R: The price of sex-role deviance: it costs men less. Paper presented at the annual meeting of the American Psychological Association, Montreal, Quebec, September 1980

Parlee MB: Psychology: review/essay. Signs 1:119–138, 1975

Parry G: Paid employment, life events, social support, and mental health in working-class mothers. J Health Soc Behav 27:193–208, 1986

Plass JA, Hill KT: Children's achievement strategies and test performance: the role of time, pressure, evaluation anxiety, and sex. Developmental Psychology 22:31–36, 1986

Radloff LS, Rae DS: Components of the sex difference in depression, in Research in Community and Mental Health. Edited by Simmons RG. Greenwich, CT, JAI Press, 1981, pp 77–110

Rieker PP, Carmen EH (eds): The Gender Gap in Psychotherapy: Social Realities and Psychological Processes. New York, Plenum, 1984

Robins LN, Helzer JE, Weissman MM, et al: Lifetime prevalence of specific psychiatric disorders in three sites. Arch Gen Psychiatry 41:949–958, 1984

Rosenfeld S: Sex roles and societal reactions to mental illness: the labeling of "deviant" deviance. J Health Soc Behav 23:18–24, 1982

Ross CE, Huber J: Hardship and depression. J Health Soc Behav 26:312–327, 1985

Ross CE, Morowsky J, Huber J: Dividing work, sharing work, and in between: marriage patterns and depression. Am Sociol Rev 48:809–823, 1983

Ruble DN, Higgins ET: Effects of group sex composition on self presentation and sex typing. Journal of Social Issues 32:125–132, 1976

Russo NF (ed): A Women's Mental Health Agenda. Washington, DC, American Psychological Association, 1985

Russo NF, Denmark FL: Women, psychology, and public policy: selected issues. Am Psychol 39:1161–1165, 1984

Russo NF, Olmedo EL: Women's utilization of outpatient psychiatric services: some emerging priorities for rehabilitation psychologists. Rehab Psychol 28:141–155, 1983

Russo NF, Sobel SB: Sex differences in the utilization of mental health facilities. Professional Psychology 12:7–19, 1981

Shaffer DR, Johnson RD: Effects of occupational choice and sex-role preferences on the attractiveness of competent men and women. J Pers 48:505–519, 1980

Sherif CW: Bias in psychology, in The Prism of Sex: Essays in the Sociology of Knowledge. Edited by Sherman JA, Beck ET. Madison, University of Wisconsin Press, 1979

Sherif CW: Needed concepts in the study of gender identity. Psychology of Women Quarterly 6:375–398, 1982

Sherman JA: Sex-Related Cognitive Differences. Springfield, IL, Charles C Thomas, 1978

Sistrunk F, McDavid JW: Sex variable in conforming behavior. J Pers Soc Psychol 17:200–207, 1971

Sonderegger TB (ed): Psychology and Gender: Nebraska Symposium on Motivation, Vol 32. Lincoln, University of Nebraska Press, 1985

Spence JT: Gender identity and its implications for concepts of masculinity and femininity, in Psychology and Gender: Nebraska Symposium on Motivation, Vol 32. Edited by Sonderegger TB. Lincoln, University of Nebraska Press, 1985, pp 59–96

Staines GL, Pottick KJ, Fudge DA: The effects of wives' employment on husbands' job and life satisfaction. Psychology of Women Quarterly 9:419–424, 1985

Task Force on Nonsexist Research: Guidelines for Nonsexist Research. Washington, DC, American Psychological Association, Division of the Psychology of Women (35), 1983

Taylor SE, Fiske ST: Salience, attention, and attribution: top of the head phenomena, in Advances in Experimental Social Psychology, Vol 11. Edited by Berkowitz L. New York, Academic, 1978, pp 249–288

Walker LE (ed): Women and Mental Health Policy. Beverly Hills, CA, Sage, 1984

Warren LW, McEachren L: Psychological correlates of depressive symptomatology in adult women. J Abnorm Psychol 92:151–160, 1983

Warren LW, McEachren L: Derived identity and depressive symptomatology in women differing in marital and employment status. Psychology of Women Quarterly 9:133–144, 1985

## Chapter 6

# Gender Ideology and the Brain: Sex Differences Research

## Ruth Bleier, Ph.D.

From the time of Aristotle, who considered women as incomplete and mutilated males, to the mid-nineteenth century, neuroscientists and philosophers defined their task as that of explaining the obvious biological inferiority of woman and her condition of arrested development on the evolutionary ladder to Homo sapiens. In contrast, contemporary scientists have undertaken the task of explaining sex differences in behaviors, characteristics, and abilities. (These are really gender, not sex, differences because biological sex, as defined by reproductive/sexual organs and chromosomes, is rarely at issue.) The term *sex differences research* therefore implies a value-free, nonjudgmental search to find the "truth" about difference. Underlying this and remaining implicit is the judgment that the "difference" considers the norm to be the white male and what is therefore difference is not merely different but inferior.

In the 1970s and 1980s, the language and theoretical commitment of many scientists to civil rights, equal rights, and equal opportunity modified the explicit ideology of female inferiority to an ideology that recognizes innate differences in personality, abilities, and aspirations and implicitly justifies the differences in life opportunities for women. Science is thus asked to provide biological and "natural" explanations for inequalities that actually have important economic, political, social, and ideological origins.

In recent years there has been intense interest in finding gender differences in brain structure and function to explain presumed gender-related differences in cognitive ability. The focus of inquiry has been mainly on the question of hemispheric lateralization of cognitive functions, particularly the processing of visuospatial information. Visuospatial ability is seen as especially critical for success in science, mathematics, and engineering, areas that have been and are still considered male domains. The dominant theory holds that males process visuospatial information predominantly with the right hemisphere of the brain, while females use both hemispheres more symmetrically.

In this chapter, I examine the premises, methods, and interpretations of recent studies purporting to provide evidence for a biological basis for these presumed differences between women and men. I also suggest the degree to which gender ideologies and stereotypes bolster a paradigm of brain dimorphism for which convincing evidence is still lacking.

## A History of Ideological Commitment

Before accepting any research finding of gender-associated differences in brain structure of cognitive function, one must maintain the highest level of skepticism, particularly in view of the history of directly contradictory findings by equally respected investigators. As Steven Jay Gould (1981) and others have documented, brain research in leading mid-nineteenth century laboratories was devoted to finding measurable differences in the structure of the brain to explain the inferior status and achievements of women and blacks compared with those of white men. Gould analyzes the manipulations of data and the convoluted interpretations by which scientists such as Paul Broca and Carl Vogt attempted to establish the inferiority of the brains of blacks and women. Vogt noted in 1864, "By its rounded apex and less developed posterior lobe the Negro brain resembles that of our children, and by the protuberance of the parietal lobe, that of our females (Gould 1981, p. 103). Broca observed in 1861, "We are therefore permitted to suppose that the relatively small size of the female brain depends in part upon her physical inferiority and in part on her intellectual inferiority" (Gould 1981, p. 104). Gustave LeBon, whom Gould considers to be the chief misogynist of Broca's school, wrote in 1879:

> In the most intelligent races, as among the Parisians, there are a large number of women whose brains are closer in size to those of

gorillas than to the most developed male brains. This inferiority is so obvious that no one can contest it for a moment; only its degree is worth discussion. All psychologists who have studied the intelligence of women, as well as poets and novelists, recognize today that they represent the most inferior forms of human evolution and that they are closer to children and savages than to an adult, civilized man. They excel in fickleness, inconstancy, absence of thought and logic, and incapacity to reason. Without doubt, there exist some distinguished women, very superior to the average man, but they are as exceptional as the birth of any monstrosity, as, for example, of a gorilla with two heads; consequently, we may neglect them entirely. (Gould 1981, pp. 104–105)

It is tempting to dismiss the science of a century ago as naive, simplistic, unsophisticated, and even ludicrous. We tend to see the scientific truths of today as the final valid truths, the culmination of primitive follies and approximations of the previous centuries. But today's truths are as contingent, as changing, and as certain to be superseded in coming decades as scientific truths were in the past.

## Contemporary Examples

A recent example of this relativity in a politically charged scientific issue lies very close to hand: the question of the size and shape of the corpus callosum. In 1982, de Lacoste-Utamsing and Holloway reported the splenium of women to be larger and more bulbous than that of men; they considered this to be important evidence of a biological basis for gender differences in hemispheric lateralization of visuospatial cognitive processing, a subject currently under investigation. Witelson (1985a) stated her commitment to the importance of constitutional factors to sex differences in behavior and cognition at a time when the study by de Lacoste-Utamsing and Holloway was the only report of a sex difference in human brain structure.

Witelson (1985a) carefully measured the corpus callosum in 42 subjects to investigate a possible correlation between hand preference and size or shape of the callosum. She included gender as a variable in her analysis and found no sex differences in the splenium, thus contradicting the de Lacoste-Utamsing and Holloway study. In addition to Witelson's report, three other studies have failed to confirm the finding of a gender-related difference in the splenium (Bleier et al. 1986; Demeter et al. 1985; Weber and Weis 1986). The finding of de Lacoste-Utamsing and Holloway, however, is now entrenched in the neuroscience literature as a fact (e.g., Kelly 1985) and will likely remain so for at least 10 years. Witelson did, however, find that the corpus callosum was larger in left-handed and ambidextrous people than in those with consistent right-handed preference. But within the year, another group investigated the relationship between the corpus callosum and handedness in 79 subjects using magnetic resonance images and found that the callosum was not larger in left-handed persons (Nasrallah et al. 1986).

What are we to make of such contradictions among well-respected investigators? There are, of course, always methodological differences among studies, but one would assume that measuring the size of a structure is a relatively straightforward procedure. Clearly it is not. This set of contradictory findings serves as a warning against the overeager acceptance of any study, particularly when, through biased interpretations of its data, it claims a significance for human evolution and cognitive functioning that reaches far beyond its ability to provide.

Today, as a century ago, scientists' agendas reflect the stereotypes and biases of the time; these biases may not be conscious, but they can find expression in hidden assumptions and incomplete or biased interpretations of the scientists' findings. Because of the women's movement and women's feminist consciousness, today's language of subjectivity and desire is more sophisticated; motives are harder to discern than they were a century ago.

## The Problem of Assessing Gender Differences in Cognitive Tests

Gender differences in behaviors and cognition—in hemispheric lateralization of cognitive functions or in brain structures relevant for cognitive processes—are not clearly established and remain controversial, as an extensive critical literature documents (Alper 1985; Caplan et al. 1985; Kimball 1981; McGlone 1980). The problems are manifold, beginning with the term *sex* or *gender* differences. At issue are behaviors and characteristics associated with one gender or the other. A person's gender, however, is an arbitrary, ever-changing, socially constructed set of attributes that are culture specific and culturally generated, beginning with the appearance of the external genitalia at birth. "Not-yet-gendered newborn males and females are shaped into the kinds of personalities who will want to perform characteristic masculine and feminine activities" (Harding 1986, pp. 147–148).[1] The expectations, demands, teachings, and rewards of parents and others shape a set of behaviors, characteristics, self-definitions, and self-expectations specified and certified as "appropriate" for one or the other gender. Yet these behaviors and characteristics themselves are what constitute, construct, and define gender; they do not result from some mystical entity or innate drive or tendency called gender.[2]

Society, having carefully constructed a set of gender characteristics to be quite specifically and normatively different for girls and boys and men and women, ingeniously observes, through its scientists, that there are "sex differences" and sets about assiduously to measure them and to find biological bases for them in our genes, hormones, or brain structures.[3]

As Kessler and McKenna (1978, pp. 162–163) carefully and insightfully explain, the social construction of gender and the everyday process of gender attribution are a part of reality construction. Scientists bring these constructions into their laboratories where they then "find" and measure gender characteristics and differences. Gender consists of a society's methods for attributing and constructing sexual differentiation. Part of that construction involves seeing gender as inevitably grounded in biology: we construct our reality in such a way that biology we think of as the ultimate truth. But gender attribution and construction can be understood as the primary process; gender is the practical outcome: we think we are discovering or confirming biological, psychological, and social differences. Actually, this arises from our focus on two genders.

The second major problem in the enterprise of finding biological bases in the brain for presumed gender differences in cognitive abilities or in hemispheric lateralization of cognitive processes is that the existence of such differences is questionable and highly controversial. The reviews noted above document that the body of literature on gender differences in spatial ability is seriously flawed by findings of marginal, if any, statistical significance; by conflicting results and failures of replication; by poor experimental design and a lack of sufficient controls for variables; and by a lack of consensus in defining the term *spatial ability*. There is little evidence that spatial ability is a unitary skill rather than a complex of elements; there is no demonstration of what the myriad tests of spatial ability are actually testing or of their relationship to each other (Caplan et al. 1985). One investigator (MacPherson 1982) administered two measures of spatial ability to 50 male and 50 female high school students. No significant gender differences were found, and, equally important, correlational analysis comparing each individual's scores on both tests revealed that no relationship existed between the two scores for individuals.

Furthermore, as many published studies find no gender differences as those that do find them. It seems clear that a fair proportion of studies finding no gender differences are never published. Meta-analysis of a body of studies on cognitive gender differences has found that when such differences are found, they account for no more than 1–5% of the population variance, and the difference between mean scores is only one-fourth to one-half of a standard deviation (Hyde 1981). The variation within each sex is far greater than the variation between them, making the concept of gender difference virtually meaningless in relation to these cognitive measures. Gender cannot be predicted by knowing a person's score, nor can a range of scores be predicted by knowing a person's gender. In addition, those gender differences that do appear on a particular test can be eradicated in a single practice session (Caplan et al. 1985).

In his review of the literature on cognitive sex differences, Hugh Fairweather (1976, p. 267) concluded, "It must be stressed, finally, that the majority of studies reviewed here and elsewhere are both ill-thought and ill-performed. . . . We cannot pretend that we are testing a theory of sex differences, since at present none can exist." At the end of a book-length review of the literature on hemispheric laterality, M.P. Bryden (1982, p. 238), a respected leader in the field, wrote, "The literature on sex-related differences in lateralization is rife with inconsistencies. . . . To a large extent, one's conclusions rest on the choice of which studies to emphasize and which to ignore.

Another problem with conclusions from these studies is that even if gender-associated differences in hemispheric lateralization of vis-uospatial function were established, there is no evidence of a correlation between hemispheric lateralization and visuospatial ability. It may facilitate processing visuospatial information to rely on both hemispheres. Marcel Kinsbourne (1974), another leading worker in the field, suggested that interhemispheric interaction, rather than hemispheric specialization, may provide an advantage in intellectual functioning.

Particular tests of verbal, spatial, or auditory processing do reveal in particular individuals some degree of greater involvement of one hemisphere in the performance of specific tasks. However, the degree to which this is true varies significantly among individuals and is affected by a number of factors. One such factor is the individual strategy pursued for problem solving; for example, some people solve visuospatial problems by using analytical-verbal strategies and there-fore appear to use both hemispheres for visuospatial problem solving.

Another example, taken from dichotic listening tests in which different auditory information is fed into each ear, is that attentional biases and different strategies for encoding or remembering stimuli "may influence the magnitude of the laterality effect observed and may even reverse the effect under some conditions or for some people" (Bryden 1982, p. 4). The problem, as Bryden states it, is that "many of the tasks employed to assess lateral specialization actually measure a diversity of things."

Finally, it seems obvious that the finding of a predominance of one hemisphere over the other in performing a particular test under circumscribed laboratory conditions is a far cry from understanding how the brain ordinarily processes the body of information. The particular test used is but one arbitrary measure, which may be culture bound, investigator defined, incomplete, and possibly irrelevant.

Roger Sperry, who won a Nobel prize for his work on hemispheric lateralization, warned against unwarranted extrapolations from his work concerning the significance of hemispheric specialization of function (Sperry 1986, p. 12):

> One must caution in this connection that the experimentally observed polarity in right-left cognitive style is an idea in general with which it is very easy to run wild . . . it is important to remember that the two hemispheres in the normal intact brain tend regularly to function closely together as a unit and that different states of mind are apt to involve different hierarchical and organizational levels or front-back and other differentiations as well as differences in laterality.

Because we know so little about the structural and functional substrates of thinking, consciousness, intelligence, and mathematical, musical, or verbal ability, or about how and where they are organized in the cortex, there is no scientific rationale for a theory of either hemispheric lateralization of or gender differences in intellectual functioning. However, we are not wanting for studies that claim to have found the sexual dimorphism in the brain that explains presumed gender differences in some cognitive abilities.

## A Theory of Testosterone and Right Hemispheric Dominance

Geschwind and Behan (1982) reported an association between left-handedness, certain disorders of the immune system, and some developmental learning disabilities such as dyslexia and stuttering, a complex more common in boys than in girls. To explain the association of left-handedness and, it was assumed, right hemispheric dominance in boys, the authors cited a study of human fetal brains (Chi et al. 1977) reporting that two convolutions of the right hemisphere

appear 1–2 weeks earlier during fetal development than their partners on the left. Geschwind and Behan proposed that testosterone,
secreted by the fetal testes, has the effect in utero of slowing the
development of the left hemisphere, resulting in right hemispheric
dominance in males and, as Geschwind stated in a subsequent com-
mentary, in "superior right hemispheric talents, such as artistic, musical, or mathematical talent" (Kolata 1983).

However, the authors failed to mention some profound problems
with their theory: there is no evidence for such an inhibiting effect
of testosterone on cortical development; rather, like estrogen, testosterone stimulates nerve growth in vitro. It is difficult to imagine how
testosterone circulating in the bloodstream could selectively affect
not only the left hemisphere alone, but only two particular convolutions on the left side. Far more serious, however, is the failure to
mention that Chi and his colleagues specifically stated that they found
no sex differences in the 507 fetal brains they examined. That finding
alone undermines Geschwind's theory. Scientific rigor and open-
mindedness require that such a finding at least be revealed, if not
explained as a contradiction to a hypothesis.

## The Corpus Callosum and Gender Differences

A second study reported what was claimed to be the first reliable sex
difference in human brain morphology: a larger and more bulbous
splenium of the corpus callosum in females (de Lacoste-Utamsing
and Holloway 1982). Despite the fact that the study was based on
only 14 brains (9 male, 5 female) obtained at autopsy and that there
was no significant sex difference ($P = .08$) in the area of the splenium,
the authors attributed "wide-ranging implications for students of
human evolution, as well as for neuropsychologists in search of an
anatomical basis for possible gender differences in the degree of cerebral lateralization" (de Lacoste-Utamsing and Holloway 1982,
p. 1431).

There were other methodological and interpretative problems
with the study: there was no mention of how the investigators selected
the 14 brains to measure after they had made the "serendipitous"
observation, in the course of examining many brains for other purposes, of a sex difference in the splenium; nor was there any information about the age or cause of death of the subjects. Furthermore,
the authors made the assumptions, for which there is no evidence,
that the size of the splenium reflects the number of axons passing
through it and is directly related to the degree of symmetry of hemi-

spheric functioning. Thus, on the basis of a series of unsupported assumptions, the authors speculate (p. 1432) that their "results are congruent with a recent neuropsychological hypothesis that the female brain is less well lateralized—that is, manifests less hemispheric specialization—than the male brain for visuospatial functions." In addition, with the suggestive phrasing "less hemispheric specialization," the authors leave it to the reader to draw the implication that they have found the biological basis for the presumed inferiority of girls and women in visuospatial functions. That the flawed methodology of the study produced flawed results is suggested by the subsequent failure of four independent studies to confirm the finding of a gender-related dimorphism in the splenium (Bleier et al. 1986; Demeter et al. 1985; Weber and Weis 1986; Witelson 1985b).

## Conclusion

My purpose in detailing these studies is to demonstrate that flawed research not only is performed but also can be uncritically accepted because it fits a dominant paradigm. The paradigm, that there are gender differences in cognitive ability and that the bases for these may be found in developmental, structural, and functional differences in the brain, persists and perhaps grows stronger over time because it supports strong beliefs based in gender ideologies and gender stereotypes. On close and critical scrutiny, influential studies may be found to be flawed by hidden and erroneous assumptions, by omission of contradictory data, and by premature and overly conclusive interpretations of inconclusive and often trivial findings. Such studies are rapidly incorporated into the neuroscientific literature and into the public mind. However problematic and erroneous they may be, they are then used as evidence by other investigators to support their own conjectures concerning gender differences in cognitive functions and real-world achievements and status.[4]

In view of what we know about the enormous plasticity of the developing brain and the effects of environment and experience on its normal growth, as well as about the complexity and malleability of human development and ability, it is remarkable that so much intellectual energy and ingenuity is spent in the search for biological bases for gender group differences that are controversial and, at most, trivial. If the aim is only to advance our knowledge about intelligence and individual differences in cognitive abilities, it would be far more fruitful to explore the wide range of abilities within a particular group than attempt to wrest significance from the trivial differences that may emerge between gender or racial groups. It is clear that not our brains, but the cultures that our remarkable brains have created pose the limitations to our visions and potentialities.

## References

Alper JS: Sex differences in brain asymmetry: a critical analysis. Feminist Studies 11:7–37, 1985

Bleier R, Houston L, Byne W: Can the corpus callosum predict gender, age, handedness, or cognitive differences? Trends in Neurosciences 9:391–394, 1986

Bryden MP: Laterality: Functional Asymmetry in the Intact Brain. New York, Academic, 1982

Caplan PJ, MacPherson GM, Tobin P: Do sex-related differences in spatial abilities exist? Am Psychol 40:786–799, 1985

Chi JG, Dooling EC, Gilles FH: Gyral development of the human brain. Ann Neurol 1:86–93, 1977

de Lacoste-Utamsing C, Holloway RL: Sexual dimorphism in the human corpus callosum. Science 216:1431–1432, 1982

Demeter S, Ringo J, Doty RW: Sexual dimorphisms in the human corpus callosum. Abstracts of Society for Neuroscience 11:868, 1985

Fairweather H: Sex differences in cognition. Cognition 4:231–280, 1976

Geschwind N, Behan P: Left-handedness: association with immune disease, migraine, and developmental learning disorder. Proc Natl Acad Sci USA 79:5097–5100, 1982

Gould SJ: The Mismeasure of Man. New York, WW Norton, 1981

Harding S: The Science Question in Feminism. Ithaca, NY, Cornell University Press, 1986

Hyde JS: How large are cognitive gender differences? a meta-analysis using $w^2$ and d. Am Psychol 36:892–901, 1981

Kelly DD: Sexual differentiation of the nervous system, in Principals of Neural Science. Edited by Kandel ER, Schwartz JH. New York, Elsevier North-Holland, 1985, pp 771–783

Kessler S, McKenna W: Gender: An Ethnomethodological Approach. New York, John Wiley, 1978

Kimball MM: Women and science: a critique of biological theories. International Journal of Women's Studies 4:318–338, 1981

Kinsbourne M: Mechanisms of hemispheric interaction in man, in Hemispheric Cerebral Function. Edited by Kinsbourne M, Smith L. Springfield, IL, Charles C Thomas, 1974

Kolata G: Math genius may have hormonal basis. Science 222:1312, 1983

MacPherson GM: The construct validity of two tests of spatial abilities. Unpublished master's thesis, University of Toronto, Toronto, Ontario, 1982

McGlone J: Sex differences in human brain asymmetry: a critical survey. Behav Brain Sci 3:215–263, 1980

Nasrallah HA, Andreasen NC, Coffman JA, et al: The corpus callosum is not larger in left-handers. Abstracts of Society for Neuroscience 12:720, 1986
Sperry R: Consciousness, personal identity, and the divided brain, in Two Hemispheres—One Brain. Edited by Lepore MF, Ptito M, Jasper HH. New York, Alan R Liss, 1986
Weber C, Weis S: Morphometric analysis of the human corpus callosum fails to reveal sex-related differences. J Hirnforschungen 27:237–240, 1986
Witelson S: An exchange on "gender." New York Review of Books, October 24, 1985a, pp 53–54
Witelson S: The brain connection: the corpus callosum is larger in left-handers. Science 229:665–668, 1985b

## Editors' Notes

1. Biological sex is determined by genetic composition and the influence of sex hormones; it begins prenatally, but powerful cultural influences begin in the first intimate interactions with caretakers.

2. All societies construct gender categories (see Chapter 1 by Dr. LeVine).

3 See the distinctions among sex, gender, and gender role in Chapter 9 by Dr. Notman.

4. This problem is not confined to the literature in neuropsychology. For years the literature on outcome of abortions, hysterectomies, and syndromes associated with menopause contained repeated citations of original studies with faulty sample selection, poor definition of concepts, and other methodological problems, leading to erroneous conclusions that remained in the literature.

## Chapter 7

# The Acquisition of Mature Femininity

## Virginia L. Clower, M.D.

In 1933 Freud wrote (p. 135), "That is all I had to say to you about femininity. It is certainly incomplete and fragmentary and does not always sound friendly." Now, more than 50 years later, there has not been a cohesive theory to supplant Freudian concepts, although they are outmoded by knowledge of human development and contributions from ego psychology. Schafer (1974) criticized Freudian theory of the psychology of women as internally flawed. The major premise that masculine development is the model for normality is another flaw. Women are then seen as defective by definition because they do not match the model. Attempts to understand femininity that are derived from masculinity have never been satisfactory, even to Freud himself. He closed his 1933 paper by saying that his successors should examine their life experiences, look to the poets, or wait until science offers more help in understanding women.

There have been many disagreements with the original theory and suggestions for its piecemeal revision. However, new data and ideas have not yet been synthesized into any coherent hypothesis within which to examine findings from biological sciences, observation of normal females, and clinical experience.

To understand how female infants become mature women, it is necessary to conceptualize a specifically feminine course of development. This conceptualization can be derived from two fundamental

An earlier form of this work was presented at the Mahler Symposium, held in Philadelphia, Pennsylvania, on May 30, 1987.

premises: that women are genetically determined to be feminine in every stage of development, beginning with conception; and that basic femininity, in concert with the individual endowment of drives and with autonomous ego capacities, is developed, differentiated, and integrated within the special bond that the female child has with the primary object of the same gender. In this chapter, I describe one model for devising a theory of psychological development in women, cite data already accessible, offer tentative formulations, and suggest areas for further study.[1]

Reports from biological sciences, studies in neonatology, and other reports that present and develop the concept of primary femininity are omitted.[2] Therefore, I will not elaborate the proposition that a female body is the fundamental aspect of feminine ego development, as Freud stated: "The ego is first and foremost a bodily ego" (Freud 1923, p. 26). Rather, I will address the second assumption and focus on the crucial experience of female infants who proceed to differentiation in the course of maturation and interactions with female primary caretakers.

## Early Development

Weil (1978) calls the ages from 1 to 3 a way station in which neurophysiological givens are elaborated into psychological formations. In this period, as well as earlier, one can see how the child experiences and enacts behaviors from patterns that have been primitively engrammed. These patterns influence separation and individuation on the ego level and on the drive level, oral, anal, and genital psychosexual progression. Characteristic feminine development can be identified by evaluating behavior observed in children during the first 3 years and material from adults that includes conflicts from every stage in the life-cycle.

Gender is certainly not the only determinant of the mode of expression of an individual's capacities. Manifestly, there are individual differences in drive endowment as well as in ego capacities that are not directly related to gender. However, the whole development experience is affected by the child's sex because the entire transaction involves caretaking, which is different for female and male children. The girl's development will be unique because at each stage of her development she brings femaleness to the interchanges with a mother who has the same constitution. Some current data about this come from direct observation and conceptualizations by psychoanalytically oriented researchers such as Mahler et al. (1975) and Parens (1979, 1980). More data are obtained from clinical work with girls and adult women. Neither of these resources has been exploited fully. The concept of a specific developmental line for women has not been used widely, and many studies still hold to the model of masculine or undifferentiated early development.

The tremendous importance of the mother-daughter bond has long been recognized. Freud (1931) spoke of the intensity of the preoedipal attachment of the little girl to her mother. In 1975, Mahler remarked that girls have a unique developmental difficulty in that they have to identify with the mother and then have to "disidentify" from the same mother in order to solve the rapprochement conflict[3] and gain individuation. On another occasion, Mahler spoke informally of the link between mother and daughter as "very sticky" (personal communication, 1978). Lichtenstein (1961) referred to the mother's feelings about a girl that resonate with her own experience as a woman and noted that these feelings are instrumental in the girl's identity formation. The mother's identification with a girl child creates a special "adhesive" in the "sticky" relationship that has been vastly underestimated in conceptualizing psychological development in women.

Mahler's general propositions about early development and the processes of separation and individuation afford a context in which the bond between girls and mothers can be studied. Mahler uses the hyphenated term *separation-individuation* as one word. However, the intrapsychic process has two intertwined tracks that do not necessarily progress simultaneously (Mahler et al. 1975). One track is that of individuation: the emergence of intrapsychic autonomy with development of the primary autonomous ego functions such as perception, memory, cognition, and reality testing. The template for this aspect of development is constitutionally and developmentally set and is modified by experience to shape a characteristically personal ego style. Gender identity obviously contributes to this ego style. The second track is that of separation: the process of differentiating the self from the other, including distancing, boundary formation, and eventual intrapsychic disengagement from the mother that paves the way for object relationships and true autonomy.

The ideal situation is one in which acquisition of individuation parallels the development of separation. As psychological development evolves through infancy and early childhood, internalized representations of the self appear as distinct from internal representations of others. If, at about the same time, competence in the child's ego functions and enhanced aggression propel the child toward independence, there is harmonious separation and individuation.

Many facets of one's endowment and the environment interact to determine the fate of these tracks; most likely there is always some divergence between the individuation pathway and the separation track (Mahler et al. 1975). For example, children who achieve early locomotion and are prompted early to separate physically from their mothers may be confronted with a kind of premature independence before they have evolved enough psychological individuation to provide cognition and reality testing sufficient for coping with this separateness.

In other children, individuation develops well but separation lags, indicated by the state of their readiness to function as separate persons without undue anxiety. A lag in separation was seen by the Mahler group in infants with overprotective mothers. Speers and Morter (1980) describe overindividuation and underseparation in children they call pseudomature.

Neither Speers nor Mahler discusses differences in maternal attitudes toward separation of boys compared with girls, nor do their case reports spell this out. They emphasize the individual's drive endowment as instrumental in the impetus toward separation. However, as a report from the Fries group notes, boy infants who are active are considered normal, whereas girls who are not so active or aggressive are considered typically feminine (Fries and Woolf 1971). I believe there are inevitable differences in both the rate of development and the eventual outcome of the two lines of separation and individuation in boys and girls because attitudes of primary caretakers are conditioned by conscious or unconscious expectations related to the gender of the child.[4]

Conflicts inherent in the special relationship between mother and daughter are central in feminine development even though these conflicts arise in the maturation of individual abilities and experiences in other important relationships. There is infinite variety in individual patterns of development, and there are many kinds of mature feminine women. Certainly, in order to comprehend the vicissitudes of development in any one person, it is necessary to know her as an individual, not as defined by gender alone. Nevertheless, certain experiences are significant in the development of the average girl in the care of an adequate mother under ordinary circumstances. Furthermore, these experiences are probably cross-cultural because young

children in every society are in the care of mothers or mother surrogates.

Given an appropriately responsive caretaker, the healthy little
girl will have a good experience in the "symbiotic phase" during her
first year. This can be a time of intensely satisfying closeness for a
mother who identifies happily with the baby and finds special satisfaction in having a daughter.

In the "practicing phase" (Mahler's term) from about 10 to 18
months, individuation is in the forefront. There is a spurt of cognition
and upright locomotion. The child's investment in his or her own
body extends toward awareness of the outside, which is explored with
glee, but at the same time maintaining ties to the mother and re-
turning to her for comfort and reassurance. Withal, the world appears
to be exhilarating, and the child in the "practicing subphase" can
venture forth with the support of a symbiotic tie barely breached.

Individuation in girls is complicated during this subphase if the
child's particular or different drive endowment and inherent ego capacities are unrecognized or unacceptable to the caretaker, for example, if a girl is bigger, more active, or more inquisitive than is
considered normally feminine. If the child develops within the limits
of conventional environmental standards, she can be easy for a mother
to identify with and to enjoy. The mother's pleasure then strengthens
the tie between them and may lead to early imitation of the mother.
This reaffirms the already secure gender identity. Such peculiar closeness can enable good individuation, within the scope of imitation
that precedes separation and identification with the mother as a separate person. It may not actually become true identification with a
separate object.

From 16 to 18 months of age, usually until well into the second
year, children of both sexes are involved in a major conflict of normal
development. During this relatively short period of time, maturation
goes on apace. The neuromuscular system, the ego functions, and the
aggressive drive burgeon. Noticing and responding to an increasing
number of people and things bring new experience with people other
than the primary caretakers. Established sphincter control and mastery of locomotion become other elements in an emerging sense of
personal identity. Ability to form concepts and to communicate in
speech implements readiness for independence. Awareness of the anatomical differences between the sexes also appears. It further delineates the self from others to include a gender identity.

There is much for an immature ego to synthesize when the child is increasingly aware of differentiation from the mother. Mahler has described the conflict between the tendency to remain in a close bond and the thrust toward separation that is part of this phase of development. As the toddler exercises new skills and an ability to move away, he or she has an increased need for the mother to be available and to share experiences. The name given this intrapsychic to-and-fro is *rapprochement*.

There is unavoidable conflict in mother-child couples as they cope with the rapprochement crisis. It is especially taxing for both child and mother to deal with the ambivalence of a child who, at the same time, loves and hates the mother. If the mother is unable to help the toddler differentiate emotionally, because of her own ambivalence and unreadiness for separation, the child may have difficulty with boundary setting, although he or she may be adequately individuated. Some children appear to need an extra push to disengage intrapsychically and to be comfortable with perceived differentiation from the mother.

Any child may have this problem, but it seems to occur more often in girls in whom it is more likely to be considered "normal" passivity. It can constitute a developmental arrest and interfere with the final achievement of autonomy, or it may simply blur a sharp sense of separation from the mother on the way to object constancy.

Some degree of vagueness in feeling separate is a condition so frequently seen in girls and adult women who are not psychotic or borderline that it commands closer scrutiny. In extreme cases it is a source of low self-esteem and crippling inhibition of appropriate independence; more normally, however, it ensures flexibility in adaptive regression, facilitating identification, empathy, and predilection for affiliation and close human relationships. These traits often are spoken of as feminine. Too often there is an implication that having such attributes constitutes evidence for deficiency in ego or superego development. On the contrary, the ability to establish and maintain intimacy requires self-definition, the capacity for object constancy, and tolerance of regression in one's self and others. Rather than judge women by standards set for men, we need to establish meaningful criteria for assessing mature femininity. This requires a coherent model for early development of women in terms of drive, ego/superego structure, and object relationships.

These gender-related differences in the rapprochement crises of normal children have occasioned some comment. Greenson (1968) felt that boys seem better able to cope with "symbiosis anxiety" and saw identification with the father as facilitating the boy's gender identity. Mahler commented on the "different flavor of the girl's rein-volvement with the mother as compared to the boy's during the rap-prochement subphase" (Mahler et al. 1975, p. 214). With greater involvement, the girl shows a heightened ambivalence to her mother, and her basic mood has a depressive coloration. The Mahler study did not explore various components of the girl's moroseness at this time, but offers the Freudian view that she is angry and sad to discover she has no penis, a deprivation for which she blames mother. There is another more probable explanation in most cases—not every little girl persistently wants a penis, but every girl has to mourn the special closeness to her mother as maturation pushes her inexorably into separation.

Bergman (1980), writing on girls in the rapprochement subphase, assumes that to some extent separation is always felt as a loss for mother as well as daughter. She agrees with Abelin (1980), who said that a daughter may fulfill the mother's need for generational iden-tity—the double wish to be a baby and to have a baby. Clinical experience affirms that the girl child is indeed a restitution for the mother in undoing the loss of her own mother in separation. Allowing a girl to pull away may be felt as giving up her mother again as well as relinquishing the baby.

One gender-determined difference in the rapprochement sub-phase is undisputed. Awareness of the sexual distinction between male and female confronts any boy who has adequate reality testing with an irrevocable unlikeness to his mother. He must then surrender the sense of being one with a symbiotic partner who is different anatomically. Turning toward male objects for libidinal gratification and imitation of activities labeled phallic supports the disengage-ment. Masculine gender identity seems to push boys toward sepa-ration, at times even before individuation is adequate. The toddler boy is bereft if he abruptly turns away from the mother's participation in his attempts at imitation and internalization, or if the mother mistakes his excursions as readiness for separateness and prema-turely withdraws her emotional availability. Such a child may then be overseparated but underindividuated.

Perhaps such divergence is inevitable and typical of development in boys. Most cultures characterize healthy masculinity as active, assertive, independent, and devoid of sentimentality. Pathological extremes are found in men who are defensively aggressive, fearful of intimacy, and intolerant of emotion and dependence. Certainly the normal boy's relatively late acquisition of gender identity brings its own problems. Even mature men have recurrent castration anxiety;

less secure men are perennially involved in maneuvers to protect their masculinity in the conflict between regression into symbiosis and progression toward separation.

The girl comes to the rapprochement subphase profoundly different from boys in at least two crucial aspects already named: her core identity is based on early mental representations of her female body and her experience of this in relationship to female caretaking. Her gender identity is not at risk. And she has the uniquely close bond accentuated by the mother's attitudes and identification with a baby of her own gender. This is an inevitable source of conflict with the tasks of separation and individuation.

From midway in the second year, the child in rapprochement crisis displays strong attachment, concurrently seeking love and attention from the mother and expressing anger and hostile rejection. The conflict in hating the person who is at the same time the object of intense investment creates anxiety. Tantrums, outbursts of tears, provocative nagging, and diffuse irritability are symptomatic.

In the rapprochement crisis, it can be especially painful for a mother to be tormented by a small image of herself whom she has heretofore enjoyed in a companionable relationship. Every mother confronts the reactivation of early stages in her own development as she participates in each child's struggles; however, it may be easier for a mother to be objective about a toddler boy who turns away from her and expresses ambivalence. His maleness has always made him different from her, and there is no realistic alternative to letting him go. A daughter, on the other hand, is so alike that her repudiation inflicts a narcissistic injury on the mother in separation. The mother feels hurt, anger, and disappointment. The daughter then shares the hurt, resents the anger, and, with guilty conflict, fears retaliatory abandonment.

This experience is reenacted with limitless variations in women's relationships with other women. It emerges plainly in the transference/countertransference with women in treatment. Painful separation conflicts are central without any defect in reality testing or in the capacity for object constancy. Such a woman cannot be considered borderline, a diagnosis often awarded "problem" female patients. This observation is of grave importance clinically because misinterpretation of feminine behavior and fantasies eventuates in unreliable diagnoses and ineffective therapeutic procedures.

Freud (1931) thought that the earliest attachment of the girl to her mother is destined to perish because it is so intense. Apparently, the more intense, the more difficult it is for each member of the pair to separate. Management of the rapprochement crisis is the mother's responsibility, and the outcome depends, to an extent, on maternal ability to negotiate detachment from the consuming closeness without destroying an irreplaceable identification.

The following cases from published reports of two girls in the Mahler study illustrate the task (Mahler et al. 1975). Donna and Wendy both had well-attuned mothers, and the symbiotic phase was fulfilling in each case. The observers expected that neither girl would have unusual difficulty in the next developmental subphase. However, both girls had painful and prolonged rapprochement crises.

**Case 1: Donna**

Donna was a well-endowed child whose mother seemed responsive to every cue. The little girl began to mature early, but in the practicing subphase she was able to enjoy her competence. In the rapprochement subphase, she continued to have difficulty in leaving her mother to carry on her own activities, holding onto the physical closeness. Toward her mother she was demanding, coercive, very ambivalent, whining, and complaining at the least frustration. The mother was reluctant to withdraw and leave Donna to her own devices. By the end of her third year, Donna still fluctuated between independent behavior in many areas and sticking babyishly to her mother. Adequate individuation was displayed in her ability to toilet herself without help, choose her own clothes, and mother dolls. The lag in separation appeared as she drank from a bottle, wanted food in her mouth, and held onto mother in anxiety-provoking situations. In retrospect, the conclusion was that her mother was unable to give Donna the encouragement she needed to distance herself and that Donna felt and responded to her mother's unconscious doubt that she could manage alone. The mother's positive wish to keep her girl close might have been another factor.

When Donna was about 3 years old, her mother began to show impatience and irritation with Donna's clinging behavior. Donna then mobilized her independence and acted more confidently. She appeared to resume development and move into the last subphase of separation-individuation, the achievement of object constancy. Her difficult rapprochement subphase did not inevitably create a developmental arrest. As her drive and ego endowment continued to mature and because her mother's problem in separation was not persistent, she continued to differentiate and consolidate her own identity. The effect of the conflict and the solutions she found for it would later be incorporated into her character and personality.

Donna's history illustrates the dilemma of girls in whom the struggle for separation is intensified by prolonged gratifying closeness with a loving and giving mother. Female patients reenact varieties of "sticky" ties with different kinds of mothers. Some patients exhibit conditions resembling borderline states, others severe hysteria, and others what have been called infantile dependent personalities. These women are often depressed and sometimes phobic. Frequently they present problems in relationships with men. Sooner or later they talk about their mothers, daughters, and past and present surrogates. Their perceptions and recollections are distorted by unresolved ambivalence. In the transference, some manifest hostility, others are overidealizing. Many of these patients are good candidates for analysis; others respond to analytically oriented psychotherapy, enabling them to resume development toward autonomy.

## Case 2: Wendy

Wendy and her mother also had a blissful early phase. Wendy showed precocious differentiation with intensive scanning of the environment and apparent recognition of different people; she protested her mother's leaving at age 3–4 months. This was thought to be due to an innate hypersensitivity in the baby. The research team believed that this hypersensitivity interfered with her ability to exploit her ego development or the resources of the environment.

Wendy's observers suspected that no mother could shield such a child entirely and that heightened perceptions might inevitably impinge on the state of an ideal symbiotic "oneness," in Mahler's terms. This is not necessarily true. The capacity to empathize with and remain close to a sensitive infant varies with each mother's tolerance of the problem of heightened perceptions and the meaning it has for her.

One can compare this situation with the problems posed by children with infantile eczema, a hypersensitivity of skin reaction. Pediatricians say that children with infantile eczema fare better if their mothers do not think the skin problem is a serious defect or the result of poor caretaking. In one adult woman I treated, the outcome of her mother's response to her unusual sensitivity was analyzed. The patient had multiple allergies from birth, with irritable skin and hyperreactivity to light and noise. Nevertheless, she experienced her mother as soothing, able to handle the child tenderly and to tolerate fussiness without infantilizing her. The problem itself thus became a support for a state of early symbiosis and later identification with a warm caretaker.

Wendy's mother was judged by the research team to be involved and gratified with her child in the early phase. Yet, the description of her also depicted a woman who was insecure and unable to lend herself to the needs of an individuating child. She left many mothering functions to her husband, and at times she left Wendy with a baby-sitter and disappeared completely.

Not surprisingly, Wendy's early development was compromised. The development of the separation and return behavior characteristic of the practicing phase was delayed and she never had a clearly manifest rapprochement crisis. When her mother was not available, she tended to be sad and angry and to withdraw by rocking herself or hugging a teddy bear. In her third year, Wendy seemed to have an overwhelming need to remain the narcissistic baby. "She did not speak much, she did not play much, she did not relate to people much" (Mahler et al. 1975, pp. 167–168).

Wendy also strongly rejected females other than mother. Observers speculated that this came from a specifically displaced externalization of the "bad" side of the mother, an individual form of splitting on Wendy's part. Interestingly, this child was very pretty, quite sensual, and appealing to adults, especially to men. In turn she was more responsive to men, and by age 3 manifested what was called a "spurious oedipal situation" (Mahler et al. 1975, p. 166). She appeared to the observers to have an atypical separation with doubtful progress toward object constancy but "without a trace of psychosis" (p. 167).

It is easy to envision Wendy growing into one type of ostensibly mature adult woman. Clinicians meet them as mothers of disturbed children or partners in troubled marriages and less frequently seeking treatment for themselves alone. In many instances they are pretty, childishly affectionate, heterosexually active, and sensual in pseudomature relationships with men. Frequently, they profess to like men and are mistrustful and hostile toward women.

Therapists recognize that people with narcissistic character disorders have internalized self representations that are split into good and bad. Kernberg conceptualizes the pathology as an investment in a pathological self structure, one in which there is no integration of "good" and "bad" self representations into a concept incorporating both elements (Kernberg 1982). Such women have difficulty with girl children, whom they identify with their own bad self. A girl can be greedy, demanding, and hostile when she begins to move out of the symbiotic orbit. At that point, the mother is called on to be tolerant of ambivalence in the child; this tolerance is impossible if she has not mastered it for herself. Here the mother's identification with a daughter, normally a source of sustained closeness, promotes narcissistic withdrawal. The mother cannot stay engaged with the girl, allow her to be ambivalent, and literally fight out the issues of separation.

Every woman repeats conflict inherent in the unique relationship with a mother in every normal developmental crisis of the life span. How can it be otherwise? The immovable core of her sexual and personal identity is grounded in the tie to her mother. This tie guarantees capacities and predispositions for acquisition of some aspects of mature femininity. The sense of being an independent person who is unlike mother in significant ways evolves painfully with more conflict about separation. Women rework this in every stage: as they continue to develop in adolescence, as young adults leaving home and making choices of love objects and life-style, with the birth of each child, and as each child grows up. We see it in middle-aged women with dependent parents. The confusion and stress of generational identity is repeated when the mother must relinquish a daughter to be cared for herself and the daughter must lose her mother to become one.

A conviction of independence and freedom to be one's self opens many doors to satisfying experience and personal growth. But ultimately, autonomy for anyone evokes a sense of loss and alienation, the existential loneliness of parting with the close early relationship. In women this is intensified as it nourishes the deep fear of being unloved and abandoned by the mother, mingled with grief and guilt at leaving her. The unique bond is both a foundation and a potential barrier for mature femininity. Folk wisdom states it: "A son is a son till he gets him a wife; a daughter's a daughter all of her life."

## References

Abelin E: Triangulation, the role of the father and the origins of core gender identity during the rapprochement subphase, in Rapprochement: The Critical Phase of Separation-Individuation. Edited by Lax R, Burland A, Bach S. New York, Jason Aronson, 1980, pp 151–171

Bergman A: Considerations about the development of the girl during the separation-individuation process, in Early Female Development: Current Psychoanalytic Views. Edited by Mendell D. New York, Spectrum, 1980, pp 61–81

Freud S: The ego and the id (1923), in The Standard Edition of the Complete

Psychological Works of Sigmund Freud, Vol 19. Translated and edited by Strachey J. London, Hogarth Press, 1961, p 26

Freud S: Some psychical consequences of the anatomical distinction between the sexes (1925), in The Standard Edition of the Complete Psychological Works of Sigmund Freud, Vol 19. Translated and edited by Strachey J. London, Hogarth Press, 1961, pp 248–258

Freud S: Female sexuality (1931), in The Standard Edition of the Complete Psychological Works of Sigmund Freud, Vol 21. Translated and edited by Strachey J. London, Hogarth Press, 1961, pp 225–243

Freud S: Femininity (1933), in The Standard Edition of the Complete Psychological Works of Sigmund Freud, Vol 22. Translated and edited by Strachey J. London, Hogarth Press, 1964, pp 7–182

Fries M, Woolf P: The influence of constitutional complex on developmental phases, in Separation-Individuation: Essays in Honor of Margaret S. Mahler. Edited by McDevitt J, Settlage C. New York, International Universities Press, 1971, pp 274–296

Greenson R: Disidentifying from mother: its special importance for the boy. Int J Psychoanal 49:370–374, 1968

Jacobson E: The Self and the Object World. New York, International Universities Press, 1964

Kernberg O: Self, ego, affects and drives. J Am Psychoanal Assoc 30:893–919, 1982

Lichtenstein H: Identity and sexuality: a study of their interrelationship in man. J Am Psychoanal Assoc 24:3–27, 1961

Litwin D: Autonomy, a conflict for women, in Psychoanalysis and Women: Contemporary Reappraisals. Edited by Alpert J. Hillsdale, NJ, Analytic Press, 1986, p 188

Mahler M, Pine F, Berhman A: The Psychological Birth of the Human Infant. New York, Basic Books, 1975

Parens H: Developmental considerations of ambivalence. Psychoanal Study Child 34:385–420, 1979

Parens H: An exploration of the relation of instinctual drives and the symbiosis separation-individuation process. J Am Psychoanal Assoc 28:89–113, 1980

Schafer R: Problems in Freud's psychology of women. J Am Psychoanal Assoc 22:459–485, 1974

Speers R, Morter D: Overindividuation and underseparation in the pseudomature child, in Rapprochement: The Critical Subphase of Separation-Individuation. New York, Jason Aronson, 1980, pp 457–479

Stoller R: Primary femininity. J Am Psychoanal Assoc 24:59–78, 1976

Weil A: Maturational variations and genetic dynamic issues. J Am Psychoanal Assoc 26:461–491, 1978

## Editors' Notes

1. There have been significant changes in psychoanalytic theory concerning feminine development and the characteristics of femininity. Although

much recent work in related fields as well as in psychoanalysis has provided the basis for major modifications, there has not yet been a unified, cohesive new theory. Dr. Clower summarizes many of the new ideas that have been put forward and offers a beginning for new theory.

2. Primary femininity is a concept originated by Stoller (1976) to refer to femininity derived from preoedipal identification with mother; it is also preconflictual—i.e., derives not from the identification with the mother resulting from resolution of the oedipal triangle, but from early interaction of the girl's genetic potential with the relationship with caretakers and internalization of what being female means in a particular social context. See also Chapter 9, "Gender Development," by Dr. Notman.

3. See Litwin (1986).

4. These expectations influence the differential expression of drive endowment.

## Chapter 8

# Ground Rules for Marriage: Perspectives on the Pattern of an Era

**Jessie Bernard, Ph.D.**

### Preamble: Is the Glass Half Empty or Is It Half Full?

"What, if anything, has changed in the last century?" The implication of this question is sometimes "Has anything really changed?" Do we merely have a situation in which, despite efforts to improve marriage and family, "plus ça change, le plus c'est la même chose"? It is a question that receives quite opposite answers from different observers. Using exactly the same data, some conclude that marriage, and hence family, have changed for the worse and are now suffering severe and perhaps even irremediable disintegration. Others label such a point of view as mere myth. The general academic "line" seems to be that, yes, there have been some changes and as a result some things are clearly wrong about the current situation of marriage and family, but in the overall perspective it remains essentially strong; the evidence actually shows marriage and the family better in some ways than in the past. Most of the research on which these conflicting conclusions are based is statistical. In and of themselves, statistics can tell us only about trends or prevalence or incidence. What looks like a lasting change to one observer may seem a mere short-term

This chapter was originally published in Horner M (ed): *The Challenge of Change.* New York, Plenum, 1983. Copyright 1983 by Plenum Publishing Corp. Reprinted with permission.

change to another. What seems like a widespread, even revolutionary, change to one observer may be minimized by another because its incidence is relatively low. In the present discussion the research data themselves are secondary to what are called "ground rules." It is clear that these ground rules have indeed changed in the last century. Whether these changes show the glass half empty or half full is difficult to discern. Whether it is under our power to fill—or empty— it is not all clear to me. The glass may be fuller now for one member of the marriage or family but emptier for another; fuller for women in some classes, emptier for those in other classes.[1]

## The Victorian Era as a Benchmark

Stanley Coben (1975) dates the Victorian age as encompassing the years from about 1820 to 1890. Scholars, he tells us, believe that "the essentially middle class Victorian culture [of those years] in both Great Britain and the United States . . . unified all but the very top and bottom of society." During this period in both countries, "a shifting consensus prevailed among the middle class on almost every matter of importance to that group. The years 1830–1890, with a height of influence in the United States around 1870 [thus] serve as plausible points in time for explanation of this [Victorian] culture."

Victorian culture was an essentially middle-class creation made possible by the wealth industrialization was producing. It was the culture, Coben reminds us, reflected in the work of Max Weber and Sigmund Freud, a culture, as Tawney, Sombart, and Marx have shown, that developed personality and character traits "well suited to promote rapid industrial and commercial expansion." Although a large part of the thinking and research on these years has dealt with industrialization, with the marketplace, with what happened to work, to careers, to bureaucracy, to technology, the real focus of Victorians, as Coben reminds us, "lay within the family." The Victorian family was the basic, essential counterpart to industrialization.

The Victorian model for marriage and family was quite different from the model that preceded it and from the one now in the process of emerging. Nancy Cott has illuminated the conditions that ushered in the Victorian era and came increasingly to characterize it:

> The period between 1780 and 1830 was a time of wide and deep-ranging transformation, including the beginning of rapid intensive economic growth, especially in foreign commerce, agricultural productivity, and the fiscal and banking system; the start of sustained urbanization; demographic transition toward modern fertility pat-

terns; marked change toward social stratification by wealth and growing inequality in the distribution of wealth; rapid pragmatic adaptation in the law; shifts from unitary to pluralistic networks in personal association; unprecedented expansion in primary education; democratization in the political process; invention of a new language of political and social thought; and—not least—with respect to family life, the appearance of "domesticity." (Cott 1977, p. 3)

The operative word is "domesticity." For in the Victorian model the husband went forth each day to grapple with the cruel, cold— social Darwinian—world and the wife remained the "heart" of the home, generating sweetness and light to bind the wounds inflicted on the husband and to serve in general as a hovering angel. Roles were defined in conformity with that model. "To an extent never true before or since," Coben (1975) tells us, "children learned," at least in theory, "the lessons necessary for success in their society. Within the home, ideally, an aggressive 'masculine' father stood between his family and a harsh economic world, a passive, nourishing 'feminine' mother kept alive the higher values of Christian morality."

It was taken for granted that the family, like the school and church, was preparing boys for participation in the industrial enterprise and girls for marriage and motherhood, teaching them respect for authority, the virtue inherent in hard work, and other tenets of *Poor Richard's Almanac*. Not until the 1960s were young men and women to challenge this model. Only then did young men protest being trained—as it looked to them—to help corporations make more money and young women the socialization that presupposed no future beyond marriage and motherhood for them.

The life span of Victorian culture in its pristine form was little more than a century. After the 1870s it began slowly to recede. Coben (1975) finds it still surviving today, more or less intact, in some segments of the population, especially among the older and among the nonurban, but he also notes especially two periods in which, though it survived, it was nevertheless seriously challenged, namely in the post–World War I 1920s and again in the 1960s. In the 1920s, he says, "Victorianism suffered irremediable damage . . . before discouragement . . . forced discontent back into quieter channels." Since the 1960s the challenge has been even more insistent.

Coben attributes great importance to social scientists in undermining crucial Victorian tenets after World War I, including especially Ruth Benedict and Margaret Mead, the Lynds, literary intellectuals like Sinclair Lewis, and Theodore Dreiser, F. Scott Fitzgerald, and, later, the several ethnic and racial groups. These assaults were directed at several facets of Victorian culture but "probably the most devastating . . . have been delivered at that culture's most vital point: 'the home.' " For some, these assaults called forth loud hurrahs. But, Coben continues,

> Those who valued that basic unit of Victorian society watched with despair as Americans tore it apart. Parents who placed personal fulfillment above devotion to spouse and children; the consequent skyrocketing divorce rate; the rapid rise of women's proportion in the work force; children who felt closer to their peers than to their parents—all delivered shattering blows to the primary Victorian haven against the world's vicissitudes. The process was hastened by feminists . . . and by intellectuals with critiques like the Lynds' and Mead's.

This same kind of despair is echoed today.

Without minimizing the importance of the work of the social scientists and literary intellectuals in the decline of Victorian culture, recognition must be paid to other underlying forces at work. For although Coben tells us that future historians may view Victorian culture "as the first fairly successful attempt to create a cohesive industrial civilization," there was an intrinsic contradiction within its ethos between, for example, the strong work ethic which had undergirded it and belief in deferred gratification on one side and the slowly recognized need for wide consumption of the goods being produced, on the other. As Coben himself notes, the very process "of economic modernization or post-modernization . . . contributed to undermining of Victorianism . . . by creating social conditions which outmoded the very culture and personality types that had most encouraged rapid modernization." The personality and character suitable for an economy of scarcity were not suitable for an economy that was coming—one based on affluence. Thus "confidence in Victorianism eroded." It was, of course, the social critics who first made clear to us the contradictions implicit in the Victorian ethos and the actual state of affairs. Their "insidious criticism of the Victorian ethos diminished the conviction with which its formidable superstructure of institutions and behavior patterns were regarded and kept and left them more vulnerable to onslaughts by minority groups . . . most obviously among college students and middle class feminists."

This, in abbreviated form, is one historian's perspective on the rise and decline of the patterns of one era—the Victorian—as they waxed, crested, and waned. Now we stand at the point where many of the components of that era's culture have all but disintegrated if not wholly dissolved. Or at least seem to some observers to have suffered severe attrition, leaving us rudderless. Or in any event, less in certitude.

Against this overview as backdrop, the present discussion dealing with several trends in Victorian marriage takes place. The general procedure to be followed is straightforward. Several ground rules of Victorian marriage are examined from the heyday of the Victorian era about a century ago up to the present in an attempt to determine "what, if anything, has changed and to assess these changing social indicators from a prospective as well as retrospective point of view," as the charge to the authors of this volume [*The Challenge of Change*] was framed.

The ground rules examined here may be encapsulated as follows:

1. Woman's place is in the home.
2. The husband is head of the household.
3. The marital bond is permanent.
4. Lifelong fidelity, or sexual exclusivity, is enjoined.
5. Parenthood is a major component of marriage.

There was an almost inexhaustible literature of sermons, polemics, etiquette books, didactic treatises, and tracts extending, elaborating, and interpreting these ground rules as well as a considerable corpus of novels showing them in operation, and interminable exegesis on all of this work. Together the rules constituted a coherent, consistent entity. For a while they seemed to work.

## Ground Rule Number One: Woman's Place Is in the Home

The term "woman's place" is almost a code word encompassing a whole sex-role ideology, the very essence of marriage in Victorian culture. In fact it might be said to include all the other ground rules as corollaries. It prescribed both the correct or proper division of labor between the sexes and the correct or proper specialization of functions between them. It implied separate, even segregated, worlds for the two sexes. There is a growing literature on the resulting "women's sphere" and "the cult of domesticity" and "the cult of true womanhood," which describes and analyzes women's place in Victorian culture (Cott 1977; Kraditor 1968; Sklar 1973) and some of its concomitants and consequences, among them the economic dependency on husbands it involved. For the corollary or counterpart to woman's place in the home was the husband's place in the work force. He was obligated to support her.

Although ground rule number one said woman's place was in the home, it did not say that it was exclusively in the home, that she was to be restricted within a kind of purdah. In practice it meant in effect primarily that she was to keep out of the labor force. She was not to "work." There were in fact quite a lot of acceptable places for a married woman provided she did not aspire to independence. So long as married women did not challenge husbands or deprive them of their services, they were permitted a tether not quite so short as the code word implied. For purely alliterative purposes, married women's permitted places can be encapsulated as the five Cs: church, community, charity, consumption, and culture. A sixth C—career— is not included because if women chose a career the ground rule precluded marriage altogether.

The first two Cs—church and community—do not call for much discussion. Even the reactionary Germans included *Kirche* as well as *Kinder* and *Küchen*, and Victorians recognized the local neighborhood also as suitable places for married women. More interesting among women's places—and ultimately more dysfunctional for them—was the consumer market. For toward the end of the nineteenth century a new phenomenon was beginning to attract the attention of social observers, namely, the emergence of a class of women who had "no duties to discharge in providing for themselves or their children" (Thwing and Thwing 1887, p. 120). Woman's place in the home was, as Charlotte Perkins Gilman (1898/1966) put it, becoming increasingly to "wait upon" the bric-a-brac with which she had surrounded herself (p. 257), for as technology relieved married women from much of the hard manual physical work of the household, many chose to elaborate their living standards rather than save their energies (Folsom 1934). As Veblen (1899/1953) noted, "conspicuous" consumption was one of the functions of middle- and upper-class married women. Arthur Schlesinger (1946) has traced the trend toward this consumer role back to the burst of affluence that followed the Civil War when the families of the newly created class of millionaires began to import European standards of elegance. Gradually the patterns filtered down to the middle and even the working classes (Schlesinger 1946). Finally the role of wife even among the least affluent came to include a large component of conspicuous consumption (Myrdal and Klein 1956). There was considerable lip-clicking among those who believed that "when those who can ill afford [even] alpaca persist in arraying themselves in silk . . . the matter is a sad one" (Schlesinger 1946, p. 40).

Sad in more ways than one. For though economists might view such emphasis on consumption as performing an important societal function (Galbraith 1973), it had deteriorating effects on married women themselves. They were ensconced in "gilded cages" which greatly increased their dependency. Charlotte Perkins Gilman (1898/ 1966) was not the only one to point this out. The Thwings, for example, in 1887 did so also (pp. 120–121):

> By one of those strange paradoxes so common in society, the idea of the subordination of women, which once made her the drudge and slave of man, now makes her the petted object of his labor and care. She is his, but not to work for him, but to be worked for. Even language shows the disposition to convert the woman and wife into the lady. We no longer have the housewife. She has been lost in the lady of the house. . . . Under conditions of equality the woman whose husband labors will not expect to be supported without labor. The large (and increasingly large) class of wives, childless, and with no home but a boardinghouse, who contribute nothing of material, intellectual, or moral wealth either in society or the family will be forced by public opinion to justify their existence.

In 1887 this was a radical challenge to ground rule number one. Married women were being challenged to contribute something material, intellectual, or moral to society or to their families.

If conspicuous consumption could have deleterious effects on married women, vicarious leisures—Veblen's other conceptualized function—could have positive ones. Since husbands were themselves too busy making money—as even Tocqueville (1840) had noted—to engage in leisure-class activities, wives did it for them (Cohn 1943). European observers came to view affluent women in the United States as the only remaining leisure class (Cohn 1943). Among working-class women, just remaining at home was enough; such leisure at least validated her husband's ability to provide for his family (Myrdal and Klein 1956). But vicarious leisure could also be performed outside the home, and it did in fact become a way of extending married women's place beyond the walls of the household.

Although the women's culture-club movement in the late nineteenth century became almost a craze (Harland and Van de Water 1905), it did create for married women an autonomous place outside the home. In some cases there was even a physical clubhouse that served as a haven for members, where women could supply support for one another in a way acceptable to their society but without violating ground rule number one. And more important, unlike the first three Cs this one had implications for autonomy. For practice in organizing made it possible for some of them—and increasingly—to move beyond the cultural toward even broader goals, to expand women's place further. Such practice could have an impact on the larger world, ultimately even on the political world.

The fifth C—charity—was also an outgrowth of the vicarious leisure made possible for married women by affluence. They had time to serve on boards of community charitable agencies (Berg 1978) as well as of such cultural institutions as orchestras, art galleries, museums, and the like. Less affluent women could perform vicarious leisure functions as volunteers in community service agencies. Still others could show the world that their husbands could support them by giving time to humbler charitable activities through church organizations. It was to take a long time until women learned that these activities had marketable value.

Ground rule number one had two quite contradictory aspects. On one side it came to make for serious mental health difficulties in women in the home, but on the other it also permitted women to be more humane in their opinions and attitudes outside the home. There is research support for both of these aspects. In the late nineteenth century there was already beginning to be discussion of the deteriorating effect that affluence was having on women. In the 1920s the "nervous housewife" was already a topic of concern (Myerson 1929). As late as 1963 Betty Friedan had spoken of the malaise she found in suburban housewives, a problem that had no name. In the 1970s researchers were beginning to pinpoint the factors involved in the housewife's poor mental health (Bernard 1972). Building on Seligman's (1974) theory of learned helplessness and the work of Lenore Radloff (1975), Marcia Guttentag concluded that the greater vulnerability to depression among women as compared to men had a dependency-related basis (Guttentag and Salasin 1976). A considerable component in the helplessness and powerlessness of housewives was related to their economic dependence. On the other hand the fact that women in the Victorian model were supported by their husbands put them in effect "above the battle." The voting records of women in political positions and public opinion polls do show that women have tended to be on the more humane side of most social issues (Constantini and Craik 1972; Fritchey 1977; Harris Poll 1972; McCormack 1975).

It was not until the second quarter of the twentieth century that ground rule number one, the very keystone of the Victorian model, buckled. During the Depression of the 1930s married women could often get jobs more easily than their husbands; during World War II they were actively recruited into the labor force; during inflationary times their incomes were needed by the family. The ramifications for marriage are widespread. Although the labor force is now recognized as a legitimate place for a married woman, her place still remains in the home as well, in the sense that she is still responsible for its operation. And the hundreds of thousands of women who wish to remain in the home, sheltered, protected, and taken care of, protest against the low status of the housewife; some feel threatened and deprived of their security.

In urban studies it has been found that when a certain proportion of the houses of a given area are taken over by an incoming group, it tends to "tip" in their direction. Analogously, when half of a population accepts a given norm, we might also speak of "tipping." Such tipping was reached with respect to the first ground rule by the 1980s when more than half of all women living with their husbands were in the labor force. Now it was the nonemployed wives who became the nonconformists. The impact of wives' employment on husbands, wives, and children was great enough to warrant calling the resulting change a qualitative as well as a quantitative one. It had widely ramifying consequences. When the husband had been the sole bread-winner it had seemed logical that he should make the family decisions. Since he paid the piper he should call the tune. But when wives were also helping to pay the piper it seemed only logical that they have some say in calling the tune.

## Ground Rule Number Two: Headship of the Husband

The "cult of domesticity" referred to above was to have other fateful implications for women than those sketched above. It implied female dependency, a theme that irradiated all the ground rules of marriage. The economic interdependence which had characterized husband-wife relationships in colonial and pre-Victorian times—and which was to continue to prevail in rural life long thereafter—began to suffer attrition in Victorian culture as affluence relieved women of more and more productive activities in and around the household. As a market economy increasingly replaced a subsistence economy and as monetary transactions came to loom larger and larger, the market expanded, and the relationship between spouses became less one of economic interdependency and more one of economic dependency on the part of the wife. Though she was still contributing services, they were not, like garden produce, eggs, or textiles, salable in the local or expanding market. Victorian marriage cannot be understood without recognition of the ramifying effects of the economic dependency of married women.

In a book on *Courtship and Marriage* in 1746, far in advance of its time, Benjamin Franklin challenged the accepted view on the inequality of the sexes. He blamed men for the inadequacies attributed to women, and Schlesinger tells us, he counseled that "the husband should rule the roost only if he were the more sensible of the two" (Schlesinger 1946, pp. 8–9). Avant garde as the book was, it went through three more editions in 13 years, and in Edinburgh yet another. The more usual position in colonial times was, however, acceptance of the ground rule that gentlewomen were to render unquestioning obedience to their husbands (Schlesinger 1946). They were also to evince that "consciousness of *inferiority*, which for the sake of *order*, the all-wise author of nature manifestly intended" (Schlesinger 1946, p. 7; emphasis in the original). The ground rule was unequivocal: the husband was indisputably the head of the household. The wife owed him obedience, submission, subordination. And according to Tocqueville (1840), in the first half of the century, she submitted not only willingly but even pridefully. Catherine Beecher (1841) borrowed her apologia for the subservient status of women from Tocqueville; status differences were intrinsic in the social order and it was better to base them on sex than on class.

Scanzoni (1979) has shown the transformations of this ground rule from the early owner-property form to the head-complement form and then to the senior partner–junior partner form, each in turn mollifying the impact on women. In Victorian marriage it was perhaps in the head-complement form but, at least theoretically, not too far beyond owner-property ideas. Thwing and Thwing (1887), citing James Schouler (1921), encapsulate the law of domestic relations current in the late nineteenth century:

> The husband as the head of the household has the right to dictate the policy of the family. The wife is expected to conform to his habits, tastes, even to his eccentricities, provided her health be not seriously endangered by so doing. The husband may even restrict his wife's calling list, or forbid her from visiting her relations. The courts also sustain him in preventing her from attending the church of which she is a member. (pp. 122–123)

A vast structure of religion and law, church and state, shored up this ground rule. The apostle Paul had admonished women to subordinate themselves to their husbands; the common law viewed the wife as swallowed up in her husband. Until relatively recently the bride still promised in the marital vow to obey her husband.

What husbands and wives really did in marriage was of course often quite different. In fact the Thwings found this ground rule already anachronistic almost a century ago. It was not even then enforceable by public opinion.

> The man who should attempt to put in practice the theory of compelling or even demanding, obedience, would find little sympathy; while the wife who refused obedience would probably be fully sustained by society, if not by the courts. While preserving the form of the time-honored belief in wifely subjection, the substance has passed away. (Thwing and Thwing 1887, p. 112)

Women, to be sure, still promised to obey, but they shrugged "their shoulders with a careless laugh at the possibility of ever being asked to fulfill their promise" (p. 119). This ground rule was honored as much in the breach as in the practice.

The Thwings favored legal and institutional change in this ground rule to conform to the times. They saw women's flouting of it as both cause and consequence of the "present chaotic state of the family" (p. 112). They argued for change in the direction of equality, not in the direction of taking away the privileges of women but by adding to their responsibilities. As things were the power of women was "conceded as a compliment, as an act of chivalry, and not as a right" (p. 120). They had more rights granted as favors than society held them responsible for. But if women were granted power not as a personal concession but as a right, they could be held accountable and duties commensurate with their authority could be demanded of them (p. 120). The Thwings argued, therefore, that the structure of marriage be rebuilt "upon the complete equality of the husband and wife in the domestic relations" (p. 112). They justified their position on the basis of scriptures, justice, and expediency.

Having then argued the case for marital equality, the authors proceeded to lay down the ground rules for implementing it. For questions related to common matters they arrived essentially at Franklin's conclusion: "experience must decide to whom the decision may be more safely committed" (Thwing and Thwing 1887, p. 122). But enlightened though they might be, the Thwings were still captive of the current conceptualization of marital roles. So "in affairs regarding the relation of the family to the outside world" they arrived at the same conclusion as did Talcott Parsons and Robert Bales (1955) many decades later. The Thwings concluded that "the peculiar training of the man fits him to be the safer guide" (p. 122). But within the household such concerns "as the selection and furnishing of the house, the oversight of servants, the training of the children, the house-mother is the natural leader" (p. 122). In personal matters each should have complete freedom. Neither should dictate what friends the other may visit, what habits he or she may indulge, what private expenses each may incur. Each should control his or her own property. The wife should have complete control of her own body. Thus the theory of equality proved in effect to result in a practical validation of the status quo.

Family power relationships 100 years later are still equivocal. The actual situation that prevails today is not easy to determine. Sociologists had engaged in an orgy of research on the subject of power in the family and produced a ballooning literature dealing with it before Safilios-Rothschild (1970) punctured it and left it in considerable disarray. The ground rule still specifies at least lip service to the theory of equality but it recognizes that bona fide power may be achieved in practice by a bargaining process in which men have greater resources (Scanzoni 1979).

Much of the research on power in marriage and family has been done in connection with the quality of the relationships and here the story is equivocal, even regressive, in the last generation. An examination, that is, of the research on the relation, if any, between marital structure and criteria of well-being, however defined, shows a remarkable difference between the older and the more recent work. Thus a study of rural families published in 1930 concluded that families which in all aspects of family life exercised joint control showed up better than those in which the husband tended to dominate in most aspects of family life. Two other studies, one by Paul Popenoe (1933) and one by E. W. Burgess and Leonard Cottrell (1939), however, found that marriages in which the husband held a slight edge over the wife were more likely to be successful than others. But Terman, on the other hand, found just the reverse. He found that, "contrary to popular opinion, the wife's dominance score correlates positively instead of negatively with her husband's happiness whereas . . . dominance in the husband correlates slightly positively with his own happiness, but not with his wife's" (Terman 1938, pp. 22–23). He found no relation between difference in dominance in husband and wife and the success of the marriage.

In this earlier work when there was a balance on the side of superior power in husbands, it was only slight; in the rural families, joint control was most favorable; and in Terman's sample, dominance by the wives. In the studies of the 1960s, however, there was hardly anything worse than a family in which there was a strong mother and a weak father. Almost every psychological pathology was traceable to such a family pattern. Lip service might be paid to the variability of possible combinations in marriage but there was often an implicit—and sometimes explicit—lesson that the best pattern was one in which there was a superordinate husband and a subordinate wife (Westley and Epstein 1969).

With the increase in two-earner families, the support of male family headship that rested to a large extent on the husband's economic contribution eroded. The official demise of this ground rule was finally recognized April 1, 1980, when the U.S. Census Bureau substituted the term "householder" for "head of household" which it had until then automatically assigned to the husband. From now on the household itself will determine who is the householder. No doubt the designated householder in many households will continue to be a male for some time to come. Still, we seem to be moving in the direction Benjamin Franklin advocated: let the one best equipped make the decisions. When young people formulate the marriage commitment in contract form they usually specify egalitarian relationships (Weitzman 1981), and polls report an increase in such a preference in the general public (Roper 1980).

## Ground Rule Number Three: Permanence

Marriage in the Victorian model was for keeps. The marital vows specified "till death do us part." People assumed the roles of husband and wife with both a religious and a legal commitment to permanence. Thwing and Thwing state the ideal situation with respect to divorce as specified in the Victorian ambience as follows:

> The nature of the marriage state does not admit of its being the subject of experimental and temporary arrangements and fleeting partnerships. The union is, and should be, for life. It is so equally in reason, in the common sentiments of mankind, and in the teachings of religion. No married partner should desert the other, commit adultery, beat or otherwise abuse the other, or forbear to do all that is possible for the sustenance and happiness of the other and of the entire family. Figuratively speaking, the two should walk hand in hand up the steps of life and down its declivities and green slopes, then lay themselves together for the final sleep at the foot of the hill. Consequently, there should be no divorce, no divorce courts, no books on the law of divorce. (Thwing and Thwing 1887, p. 153)

Still, though the ground rule forbade divorce, provisions for it were made and already, then as now, there were cries of alarm about the rising divorce rate which was awakening "great apprehension for the perpetuity of important social institutions" (Thwing and Thwing 1887, p. 153). In New Hampshire in 1860, for example, there were 107 divorces; in 1882, 314, thus almost tripling in 22 years. In Vermont there was 1 divorce to every 23 marriage licenses granted; by 1878, 1 in every 14. In Maine in 1880, 1 to almost 10. In Connecticut the annual average rate for the 15 years after 1863 was 1 divorce to just over 10 marriages. In Massachusetts the number more than doubled between 1860 and 1878. Nor was the situation any better outside of New England. Indiana had 1 divorce for every 12 marriages in 1884; Michigan, 1 to every 13. In Cook County, Illinois, the annual rate for six years was 1 divorce to 9 marriages. In San Francisco, a divorce was reported for every 8 marriages; in 29 other counties of California a divorce was granted for every 7 licenses in 1882. Then there was Marin County:

> One county in California deserves perhaps to be called the banner divorce section of the United States. It bears the name of Marin, and has as its capital San Rafael, a snug and acceptable retreat, under the shadow of great cities, easy to flee to for the concealment or dispatch of the unseemly business. This county "reports 57 licenses, and 27 divorces"; or one divorce for every two and eleven-hundredths marriages. (Thwing and Thwing 1887, p. 155)

Whatever the actual divorce rate may be at any particular time, it always seems to be soaring. Actually in the 40 years between 1920 and 1960, with the exception of the 1946 dissolution of wartime marriages, the increase had been fairly moderate, even reaching a relatively low point in 1958.

The discussion of the causes of this shocking rise in divorce almost 100 years ago seems to validate the old cliché, "plus ça change, plus c'est la même chose."

> The last fifty years have apparently changed the marriage relations from a permanent and lifelong state to a union existing during the pleasure of the parties. The change thus swiftly wrought is so revolutionary, involving the very foundations of human society, that we must believe it to be the result not of any temporary conditions, but of causes which have been long and silently at work. (Thwing and Thwing 1887, p. 158)

Equally familiar is the Thwings' analysis of the causes: the growth of individualism; the reduction of marriage by secularization from status to a mere contract terminable at either party's pleasure or convenience; the attrition of the sacred or religious nature of marriage; the loosening of divorce laws; social mobility; affluence (Thwing and Thwing 1887, pp. 159–162). And of course, the changing status of women.

The rise in the number of divorces vis-à-vis the number of marriage licenses granted called for serious consideration. It challenged the very keystone of Victorian marriage, ground rule number one, which defined woman's place. It forced a reconsideration of the nature of the "ties that bind." The question for some became not why people leave a marriage but why they remain in it. What *are* the ties that bind: law, religion, conscience, love, duty, social sanctions, habit? Or in the case of women, need for economic support? For the current scene there is strong research evidence favoring the last answer. Cherlin (1979), for example, finds that "wives whose potential wage compared favorably with the wage of their husbands had a greater probability of dissolution" (p. 164). The increased labor force participation of women may indeed thus be a significant factor in rising divorce rates. Essentially the same conclusion was being reached almost a century ago:

> Her [a woman's] sphere of activities has broadened in every direction. In nearly every business, trade, and profession, women now appear as the competitors of men. Fifty years ago, the household and the school house marked the boundaries of the sphere of women's work. The industries in which she now engages are numbered by the hundreds. Such a radical change, made in so short a time, cannot fail to exercise disturbing effects on the family. (Thwing and Thwing 1887, pp. 162–163)

The potential independence then becoming available to women was making them less willing to remain in an unsatisfactory marriage; for if a woman "fails to find happiness, justice, and recognition of her personality in her position as wife and mother, a woman is now independent of this position, so far as the supply of her needs is concerned. Means of a decent livelihood for a competent woman open on every side" (Thwing and Thwing 1887, p. 163). So what reason was there for a woman to remain in an unsatisfactory marriage?

Education had also played into the hands of women, making them less dependent on men.

> The educational advantages for women have kept pace with their enlarged opportunities. The education of the average American woman, so far as it pertains to a knowledge of books, is undoubtedly superior to that of the average man. Especially is this true in the middle class, a class among which the rate of divorce is by far the highest. Among this class in the older groups the intellectual superiority of the wife

> to the husband is plain to even a casual observer. (Thwing and Thwing
> 1887, p. 163)

The women's colleges no doubt contributed to the "intellectual superiority" of wives.

The expanded rights accorded to women were also a contributing factor in the high divorce rates. They had been enlarged without any corresponding recognition of accompanying duties. "As an individual the rights of women are now fully recognized before the law. While her political disabilities have not been removed, save in two Territories, her rights to acquire and hold property, to carry on business, or to be a party to a suit are fully granted" (Thwing and Thwing 1887, p. 162). But the women have not risen to these challenges: "We thus find a class of irresponsible women, who, while jealous of all rights, neither hold themselves, nor are held by society, to a strict performance of duties commensurate with their rights" (Thwing and Thwing 1887, p. 165). The authors thus conclude that "the enlargement of women's rights has increased the number of divorces; and it may have already also proved a cause of dissoluteness, and have tended to disintegrate the conserving forces of the republic" (Thwing and Thwing 1887, p. 168).

The remedy? Clearly women could not be denied access to jobs, nor could their education be abridged, nor could their rights be withdrawn, nor their independence revoked. What was needed was greater emphasis by women on the duties and responsibilities imposed by their independence (Thwing and Thwing 1887).

Some 40 years later, during the recession of the Victorian ethos in the 1920s referred to by Coben (1975), a feminist interpretation of the same kinds of facts was viewing divorce not as the destruction of marriage and family but as a redress for women. Divorce was a measure not of societal breakdown but of the status of women, the higher the rate the higher their status:

> In all of these circumstances in which we are confronted with divorce
> as essentially a mode of redress for women, we are dealing with one
> partner who for the first time in history is not bound hand and foot
> in her situation. This is one of the interesting fruits of the fact that
> her serious economic value as a worker finds expression outside of
> rather than within the home. Work is no longer deeply identified
> with the tie of sex in woman's case, but is largely independent of it.
> This opens a door which does not necessarily imperil the bond of
> love and the integrity of the marriage contract but it does put it to
> the test, in that it must hold henceforth largely on its genuine merit.
> If it is spurious and not real it is no longer supported and indefinitely
> continued by the old economic organization. (Messer 1928, p. 332)

Instead of seeing divorce as a negative phenomenon, this woman saw it as a positive force. "The new order, as economically organized, enables woman's 'taste in sex to remain noble' (to borrow the fine German phrase)" (Messer 1928, p. 332). It makes for purifying and perfecting domestic life as well as for disrupting it. A similar point with respect to the selective effect of divorce was made in my paper on success in marriage (Bernard 1934), and by Veroff, Douvan, and Kulka in 1981: "In a number of ways . . . the modern institution of divorce may be a force not weakening but strengthening marriage in American Society" (p. 163). It thus also raises the status of women. The fact, then, was that a woman's "serious economic value as a worker" released her from the psychology of serfdom, from the status of a pet bred for incompetence. Liberated now from "all these states in which the old home actually found much of its security and basis, she sets up a requirement befitting a human being. And in the process she is likely to avail herself of all the help the law affords" (Messer 1928, p. 333). Including, of course, the law of divorce.

It is interesting to note how frequently divorce is discussed in connection with the position of women. Although it is true that most divorce suits are brought by women, some of them, W. J. Goode (1956) has told us, are the result of what he calls the "strategy of divorce" by which husbands manipulate wives to bring action. Actually a considerable corpus of research shows that marital dissolutions are economically bad for a large number of women, for the erosion of the general rule of permanence in marriage ramifies widely, especially among those left stranded by divorce, desertion, or abandonment after years of marriage and also among their children. Lois B. Shaw (1978) found, for example, that a fourth of white families and half of black families became poor after marital disruption.

Although the economic costs of divorce are greater for women than for men, the reverse may be true for emotional and psychological costs. Commitments to psychiatric hospitals tend to be substantially higher for divorced/separated men than for divorced/separated women (Bloom et al. 1979). But household surveys of noninstitutionalized populations show psychiatric impairment slightly higher among divorced women (42.1%) than among divorced men (40%) (Bloom et al. 1979).

We are, as a society, still wrestling with the kinds of ground rules to apply when permanence ceases to be recognized at all. How much emphasis, if any, should be placed on permanence and just how the partners, especially wives and children, can best be protected in nonpermanent relationships still waits on further research for answers. The hope is that the phenomenon of "displaced housewives" will eventually die out by attrition. It is hoped, that is, that in the training of girls it will be made clear to them that they cannot count on "being taken care of" all their lives, that the chances are not insignificant that they will be left on their own some time or other in their lives so that the "trained helplessness" which crippled so many women reared under the old ground rules will not be their fate. And also that the care of children as well as their support can be as much expected from fathers as from mothers. These goals of course presuppose the elimination of discrimination in other roles as well, at the work site as well as at home.

Whether we accept the Thwings' evaluation or Messer's, whether, that is, we see the modification in the ground rule of permanence as evidenced by divorce as bad or good, as constituting a step toward societal disintegration or a giant step forward for women, it is clear from the trends in divorce that permanence is no longer a major ground rule in marriage. Norton and Glick (1979) estimate that 4 out of every 10 marriages entered into by women born between 1945 and 1949 would eventually terminate in divorce. This is considerably higher than the estimated 3 out of 10 for women born a decade earlier (Norton and Glick 1979). The same rate of increase would lead to an expectation that half or more of marriages contracted by women born in the 1950s would end in divorce. Thus although most marriages now as in the past still conform to the ground rule prescribing permanence, enough do not as to challenge its viability. Divorce now outstrips death as the cause for marital disruption. In 1860 only 4.1% of all marital disruptions had been by divorce; in 1900, 12.5%; by 1950 the proportion had reached 36.2% (Jacobson 1959, Table 70). By 1973–1974 for the first time in our history the proportion was more than half (Glick, n.d.). Just as changes in ground rules one and two reverberated in ground rule number three, so also do changes in the ground rule of permanence have impact on ground rule number four, fidelity.

A generation ago the term "serial monogamy" was coined to refer to the situation in which men and women went from one monogamous relationship to another (Landis 1950). It was pointed out that in our country there was as much polygamy in terms of the proportion of people who engaged in it sequentially if not concomitantly as there was in societies that officially permitted it. The trend has continued until now a new marital status—"transitional"—is coming to be recognized (Ross and Sawhill 1975). Such sequential or serial polygamy is related to another ground rule which characterized Victorian marriage, namely, the rule of sexual exclusivity.

## Ground Rule Number Four: Fidelity

The ground rules of the Victorian family specified not only monogamy but also exclusivity. Not only one wife or husband throughout one's life but also only one sex partner ever, before or after marriage. Virginity before and chastity after marriage were enjoined, theoretically for both partners but both theoretically and actually for women. Monogamy was undergirded by law, exclusivity by both law and the marital vow. Adultery, a legal concept, was forbidden by both legal and religious norms. Thus engaging in sexual relations with anyone other than a spouse was both a crime and a sin. It is still universally accepted as grounds for divorce wherever divorce is granted. Infidelity, as distinguished from adultery, was violation of a promise made at marriage to "forsake all others." But the precise nature of what these promises included became murkier and murkier.

A relatively superficial examination of the literature on infidelity suggests at least seven kinds of infidelity of varying levels of seriousness: 1) coquetry and flirtation; 2) fly-by-night sex; 3) "the matinée" or playful relationship among working men and women; 4) cocktail-lounge relationships; 5) monogamous and permanent relationships outside of marriage; 6) fantasied infidelity; and 7) noncoital, nonfantasy relationships which involve intimate sharing of the self (Bernard 1972). Perhaps there should also be added the recently advocated forms of technical infidelity exemplified by such relationships as "open marriage," group marriage, some kinds of communal relationships, and swinging.

Another straw which shows which way the wind is blowing with respect to the ground rule of fidelity is the phenomenal increase in so-called swing clubs in the 1960s, 1970s, and 1980s (Bernard 1968, 1972, 1982). "Swinging," or organized spouse-sharing, has been called one of the fastest growing forms of—commercialized—recreation or entertainment in the country. On a television program early in 1982, the president of the National Association of Swing Clubs, Robert McGinley, a counseling psychologist, estimated that there were 200 "swing clubs" in the country and perhaps 5,000,000 swingers (transcript of interview, "Phil Donahue Show," January 19, 1982).

That the ground rule of exclusivity is changing may be inferred by several straws in the wind. There is, for example, increasing emphasis on the positive aspects of extramarital relationships by researchers and counselors as well as by some ethicists. There is not only tolerance but even advocacy on the part of some (Sapirstein 1948). The increasing frequency of infidelity among women is further evidence of the attrition in the rule of fidelity. The trends in divorce also suggest that fidelity is no longer conceived of as intrinsic to marriage. Despite the documented frequency of adultery, the grounds alleged for divorce have changed dramatically from a frequent use of adultery to a frequent use of cruelty. In 1938, a *Ladies Home Journal* survey reported by H.F. Pringle found that three-fourths of the respondents did not think a single act of adultery by either spouse should necessarily lead to divorce. And with the introduction of the no-fault concept of divorce, fidelity is no longer intrinsic to marriage. A person who engages in extramarital relationships but does not want a divorce cannot necessarily be divorced for this alone. Unless there are those who wish to prosecute for the crime of adultery, it will for all intents and purposes disappear as a legal entity.

A question has been raised with respect to the relationship between the ground rule of exclusivity and the ground rule of permanence. There may be an implicit conflict between the two. That is, they may be incompatible. We may have to choose between them. If we insist on permanence, exclusivity may be harder to enforce; if we insist on exclusivity, we may be endangering permanence. Exclusivity meant one thing when a marriage lasted only, let us say, about 25 years; it is another when it may last twice that long. A comparison of Kinsey's (Kinsey et al. 1953) findings and findings on young couples living together outside of marriage suggests that exclusivity is more important to the young people but permanence more important to the older couples. "The trend ... seems to be in the direction of exclusivity at the expense of permanence in the younger years but permanence at the expense of exclusivity in the later years" (Bernard 1972, pp. 113–115).

There has been only a moderate amount of exegesis on fidelity. But of considerable interest was the conclusion of two commentators that fidelity did not condone jealousy of innocent friendships. In Victorian marriage such friendships were common among women (Smith-Rosenberg 1975). But women's "place" did not foster them with men. Now that there are so many places for women outside the home, the opportunity for friendships between the sexes increases. There is an almost unlimited literature on the joy of sex. But with the increasing opportunity for contacts between men and women in a variety of settings, new kinds of "joy" become possible which are not dependent on genital relationships, such, for example, as the "joy of gender," the kind of pleasure men and women sometimes achieve in the interplay of personality, erotic perhaps but not necessarily genital. In a London play some years ago the wife was justifiably more concerned about the Platonic intimacy between her husband and another woman than she would have been about a coital relationship. For

> the kind of relationship which can develop between men and women who work together as a team over a period of time sometimes assumes an emotional interdependence outweighing the marital bonds of either one without supplanting them. These may be among the innocent relationship . . . not forbidden by the marital vows. (Bernard 1972, p. 107)

There is as yet little research on this kind of relationship and it is only now beginning to attract attention as the potential reaction of wives to having their husbands work closely with female professional colleagues becomes a factor in women's careers.

Both exclusivity and permanence as ground rules for marriage have been subjected to a considerable research scrutiny in the recent past, especially vis-à-vis the so-called sexual revolution and alternate life-styles. Many marriages still conform at least moderately well to both rules. But increasing numbers seem not to be conforming to either one. A vast body of experience is being accumulated related to nonconformity to both of them. Precisely what is the degree of exclusivity that should be incorporated in the ground rules of marriage to produce, overall, the least amount of suffering and the most benefit to both partners is something we will only know as more definitive research is available.

## Ground Rule Number Five: Bear Children

Because it introduces a totally different realm of discourse—the demographic—only a bow is made here in the direction of another, quasi-ground rule of Victorian marriage: bear children. It is qualified by the term "quasi" because although there was no ground rule more basic, more unchallenged, more taken-for-granted, compliance was not always possible. A couple might be pitied if they could not conform but they could not be sanctioned. This rule had scriptural foundations so unequivocal that legal support was not necessary except in the form of prohibiting contraception and punishment for abortion. It seemed to have been laid down by Nature herself in the form of a maternal instinct or at least of mother love. Still, Nature was not wholly relied upon; powerful pressures were invoked, just in case Nature did not succeed (Bernard 1974). But in recent years the whole environmental and ecological movement has counteracted these pressures with negative ones. Thus in a Gallup poll in 1975 1 parent in 10 said that if they had it to do over again they would have no children, a 10-fold increase over the results of a similar poll 10 years earlier (McLaughlin 1975). And an increasing—though admittedly still small—number of young couples do indeed report that they plan to have no children at all (Veevers 1979). The creation of a National Organization for Optional Parenthood with chapters all over the country highlights the revolutionary change in this ground rule. The proportion of women who say they want no children remains small, although it may be increasing. It was 1.3% among those 18–24 in 1967 and 3.9% 4 years later (Bernard 1974). In two surveys, 1957 and 1976, it was found that there had been "a 5 percent rise in childlessness for the youngest age group who were married at one time or another" but this did not necessarily imply a "new norm against having children" (Veroff et al. 1981, p. 198).

A corollary in Victorian marriage to the ground rule to bear children was the rule that child care was the sole responsibility of women. Here too change is in process. Thus rearing children is becoming the first choice of a smaller and smaller proportion of women. A Louis Harris Survey in 1975, for example, found that "the percentage of women who believe that 'taking care of home and raising children is more rewarding for women than having a job' has declined from 71% to 51% in the past five years." Child care may prove to be the most intractable aspect of marriage to find new consensual ground rules (Bernard 1976a).

## Whither Bound?

This retrospective sketch shows that in answer to the question raised earlier, a great many things about marriage and family have indeed changed since the founding of Radcliffe College a century ago. Although the "place" of women is still in the home, it is not the only place for them; there are a great many other places for women. Although equality of status within the household is not yet achieved, some headway, especially among the young, seems to be in process. Although most marriages—some 60%—are still lifelong in duration, and although permanence may be the dream of young lovers, it is no longer taken for granted. Lifelong fidelity, like permanence, may also be the dream of young lovers, but no more than permanence is it taken for granted. Pressures to have children still remain strong, but support for those who choose not to is also becoming strong.

It is far easier to point to past forms that are disintegrating than it is to discern prospectively the new forms in process of emerging. Or to delineate the new forms to aim for. Or to be sure how to create them. Or just how much we can actually control them. There is a perennial controversy in the literature of jurisprudence and sociology with respect to the limits of change that can be achieved by way of law. Those who have looked on the ground rules of marriage as established by Divinity or by Natural Law and as supported by reason and human nature or by "biogrammer," find that law and legislation can do little to change them. In the nineteenth century this was a commonly expressed view; it still is today. Thus some students doubt whether "changing attitudes and even laws will induce people to act in ways that contravene, contradict, or distort what may be natural mammalian patterns" (Tiger and Shepher 1975, pp. 12–13). If we knew what were the "natural mammalian patterns" that neither attitudes nor laws can change, it would greatly help us in planning for the future.

Sometimes collective behavior changes and law belatedly catches up with it; more rarely law changes and collective behavior changes to conform (Bernard 1942, 1976b). In the case of marriage the first pattern seems to be more common. Thus, for example, divorce by collusion was being granted long before no-fault divorce laws rendered it unnecessary. Or the law is nullified in effect by not imposing sanctions for violation. The crime of adultery, for example, is almost never prosecuted and is rarely anymore even a ground for divorce. The legal obligation of husbands and fathers to support their families is flouted by thousands of men without enforcement by the courts. The spread of alternative styles of relationships which involve technical adultery or extramarital relationships is not stopped by the enforcement of the law against them.

The problem is even more complicated when we turn to the indirect effect of law on marriage, such as the effect of laws dealing with property rights, with taxes, with credit, and the like. It usually takes a considerable amount of research to tease out all the indirect effects of any legislation. Tax laws, for example, may encourage marriage or discourage it, may help or hinder labor force participation by wives and mothers, may encourage or discourage having the extra child. Welfare laws may encourage men to desert their families (Moles 1979). So aware are we becoming of these indirect effects of legislation on marital roles that "family impact" statements are being asked for to accompany all federal programs, just as an environmental impact statement is asked for in other kinds of legislation.

Law will be involved in a host of changes now being proposed. Contractual marriages, for example, will have to be sanctioned by law if they are put to the test. Marriage between homosexuals will also call for legal validation. In almost all the viable alternative lifestyles where property is seriously involved there will have to be legal support. The most controversial interface between marital relations and the law has to do with constitutional guarantees of equality. If such equality could be incorporated in the Constitution, the effect would be to codify the emerging ground rules of marriage and bring old ones up to date. It would not, in and of itself, change them, but it would help us in clarifying them. No demand could be legitimized for one sex that was not also legitimized for the other. The actual implementation of the ground rules would still have to be worked out between the marital partners. Such guaranteed legal equalization could not change the fact that there are a variety of functions that have to be performed in any social system—that people have to be fed, for example, and children cared for—but the arbitrary assignment in all cases of any specific function to any individual solely on the basis of sex would not be shored up by law.

These then were the ground rules for marriage when Radcliffe began its first century. And these were the events which transformed them during that century. What they will be at the second centennial is not at all clear at this moment. But it is certain that Radcliffe, through the research it fosters, through the standards it projects, through the women scholars it nurtures, will have a great deal to do with the form they will take.

## References

Beecher C: Treatise on Political Economy. New York, Harper & Row, 1841

Berg BJ: The Remembered Gate, Origins of American Feminism: The Women and the City 1800–1860. New York, Oxford University Press, 1978

Bernard J: Factors in the distribution of success in marriage. American Journal of Sociology 40:49–60, 1934

Bernard J: American Family Behavior. New York, Harper & Row, 1942

Bernard J: Present demographic trends and structural outcomes in family life today, in Marriage and Family Counseling. Edited by Peterson A. New York, Association Press, 1968

Bernard J: Infidelity: some moral and social issues, in Science and Psychoanalysis, Vol 16. Edited by Masserman JW. New York, Grune & Stratton, 1972

Bernard J: The Future of Motherhood. New York, Dial, 1974

Bernard J: Women, Wives, Mothers. Chicago, IL, Aldine, 1976a

Bernard J: Change and stability in sex-role norms and behavior. Journal of Social Issues 32:207–223, 1976b

Bernard J: The Future of Marriage (Offset Edition). New Haven, CT, Yale University Press, 1982

Bishop JP: New Commentaries on Marriage, Divorce, and Separation. Chicago, IL, TH Flood, 1891

Bloom BL, White SW, Asher SJ: Marital disruption as a stressful life event, in Divorce and Separation, Context, Causes and Consequences. Edited by Levinger G, Moles O. New York, Basic Books, 1979

Burgess EW, Cottrell LS: Predicting Success or Failure in Marriage. Englewood Cliffs, NJ, Prentice-Hall, 1939

Cherlin A: Work life and marital dissolution, in Divorce and Separation, Context, Causes and Consequences. Edited by Levinger G, Moles O. New York, Basic Books, 1979

Coben S: The Assault on American Victorian Culture. New York, Oxford University Press, 1975

Cohn DL: Love in America. New York, Simon & Schuster, 1943

Constantini E, Craik KH: Women as politicians: the social background, personality and political careers of female party leaders, in New Perspectives on Women. Edited by Shuch-Mednick M, Schwartz S. Journal of Social Issues 28:217–236, 1972

Cott N: The Bonds of Womanhood. New Haven, CT, Yale University Press, 1977

Folsom JK: The Family and Democratic Society. New York, John Wiley, 1934

Franklin B: Courtship and Marriage, 1746

Friedan B: The Feminine Mystique. New York, WW Norton, 1963

Fritchey C: The true champions of family life. Washington Post, December 3, 1977

Galbraith JK: Economics of the American housewife. Atlantic Monthly 232:78–83, 1973

Gallup Poll, 1975

Gilman CP: Women and Economics. New York, Harper Torchbooks, 1966 (Originally published, 1898)

Glick PC: Remarriage: some recent changes and variations. Unpublished manuscript, no date (Available from author)

Goode WJ: After Divorce. New York, Free Press, 1956

Guttentag M, Salasin S: Sex differences in the utilization of public supported health facilities: the puzzle of depression. Unpublished manuscript, Harvard University, 1976

Harland M, Van de Water V: Everyday Etiquette. Indianapolis, IN, Bobbs-Merrill, 1905

Harris Poll, 1972

Harris Survey. Washington Post, December 14, 1975

Jacobs AC, Angell R: A Research in Family Law. (No publisher given), 1930

Jacobson PH: American Marriage and Divorce. New York, Rinehart, 1959

Kinsey AC, Pomeroy WB, Martin CE, et al: Sexual Behavior in the Human Female. Philadelphia, PA, WB Saunders, 1953

Kraditor AS (ed): Up From the Pedestal. Chicago, IL, Quadrangle, 1968

Landis P: Sequential marriage. Journal of Home Economics, 42, 1950

McCormack T: Toward a nonsexist perspective on social and political change, in Another Voice: Feminist Perspectives on Social Life and Social Science. Edited by Millman M, Hanter R. New York, Anchor, 1975

McLaughlin M: Parents who wouldn't do it again. McCall's 103(2):37–38, 1975

Messer MB: The Family in the Making. New York, Putnam, 1928

Meyerson A: The Nervous Housewife. New York, Little, Brown, 1929

Moles O: Marital dissolution and public assistance payments, in Divorce and Separation, Context, Causes and Consequences. Edited by Levinger G, Moles O. New York, Basic Books, 1979

Myrdal A, Klein V: Women's Two Roles. London, Routledge & Kegan Paul, 1956

Norton AJ, Glick PC: Marital instability in America: past, present and future, in Divorce and Separation, Contexts, Causes and Consequences. Edited by Levinger G, Moles O. New York, Basic Books, 1979

Parsons T, Bales R: Family, Socialization, and Social Process. New York, Free Press, 1955

Popenoe P: Can the family have two heads? Sociology and Social Research, September–October 1933, 18, QS GS

Pringle HF: What do the women of America think? Ladies Home Journal, February 1938

Radloff L: Sex differences in depression: the effects of occupation and marital status. Sex Roles 1:249–265, 1975

Radloff L: Demographic groups by average CES-D (depression) score: all . . . whites only. Unpublished manuscript, July 1976 (Available from author)

Roper Organization: The 1980 Virginia Slims American women's opinion poll, 1980

Ross H, Sawhill I: Time of Transition. Washington, DC, Urban Institute, 1975

Rossi A: A biosocial perspective on parenting. Daedalus 106(2):1–31, 1977

Safilios-Rothschild C: The study of family power structure: a review 1960–1969. Journal of Marriage and the Family 32:539–552, 1970

Sapirstein MR: Emotional Security. New York, Crown, 1948

Scanzoni J: An historical perspective on husband-wife bargaining power and marital dissolution, in Divorce and Separation, Conditions, Causes and Consequences. Edited by Levinger G, Moles O. New York, Basic Books, 1979

Schlesinger AM: Learning how to behave, in A Historical Study of American Etiquette Books. New York, Macmillan, 1946

Schouler J: A Treatise on the Law of Marriage, Divorce, Separation and Domestic Relations. Cited in Domestic Relations, Vol 1. Albany, NY, M Bender, 1921, pp 122–123

Seligman MEP: Depression and learned helplessness, in The Psychology of Depression: Contemporary Theory and Research. Edited by Friedman RJ, Katz MM. Washington, DC, Winston & Sons, 1974

Shaw LB: Economic consequences of marital disruption. Unpublished manuscript, 1978

Sklar KK: Catherine Beecher: A Study of American Domesticity. New Haven, CT, Yale University Press, 1973

Smith-Rosenberg C: The female world of love and ritual: relations between women in nineteenth century America. Signs 1:1–30, 1975

Terman L: Psychological Factors in Marital Happiness. New York, McGraw-Hill, 1938

Thwing CF, Thwing CFB: The Family, An Historical and Social Study. Boston, MA, Lee & Shepard, 1887

Tiger L, Shepher J: Women in the Kibbutz. New York, Harcourt Brace Jovanovich, 1975

Tocqueville A de: Democracy in America, Part Two: The Social Influence of Democracy. New York, Langley, 1840

Veblen T: The Theory of the Leisure Class. New York, New American Library, 1953 (Originally published, 1899)

Veevers JE: Voluntary childlessness: a review of issues and evidence. Journal of Marriage and the Family 2(2):1–26, 1979

Veroff J, Douvan E, Kulka RA: The Inner American, a Self-portrait From 1957 to 1976. New York, Basic Books, 1981

Weitzman LJ: The Marriage Contract, Spouses, Lovers, and the Law. New York, Free Press, 1981

Westley WA, Epstein NB: Silent Majority. San Francisco, CA, Jossey-Bass, 1969

## Editors' Note

1. Dr. Jessie Bernard published her ground-breaking work, *The Future of Marriage*, in 1982. In this chapter, which first appeared in *The Challenge of Change* (1983), she discusses the evolution of views and basic assumptions about marriage that have changed. She challenges previous assumptions and describes the sources of shifts in expectations. Although the patterns of marriage have continued to change, especially with the increase in dual-career families, single heads of households (predominantly women), commuting marriages, and the impact of the AIDS epidemic in affecting sexual freedom and experimentation, this chapter remains an important statement in the analysis of marriage.

*Chapter 9*

# Gender Development

## Malkah T. Notman, M.D.

In recent years, traditional theories of the psychology of women have been reconsidered and questions have been raised about the basis of sex role differentiation and definitions of traits, attitudes, and characteristics that are labeled masculine and feminine. Although we recognize that complex psychological and biological differences exist between men and women, the etiology, implications, or extent of many of these differences is not clear. What has become more apparent is that the enormous and overlapping range of attributes and behaviors that are within the "normal" range for both men and women occupies a very important role. The enormous impact of socialization has also been recognized. Influences from the environment combine with genetic determinants from the very beginning.

Psychoanalytic theory has also changed in many areas as evidenced by a variety of sources, including information from biology, sociology, and the impact of data from direct observations (Alpert 1986; Bernay and Cantor 1986; Notman 1982). In this introduction to feminine development, I present a number of older views and the changes that have evolved as new data have emerged.

Recent thinking has emphasized that in many areas there are separate developmental paths for males and females (Clower 1987; Tyson 1982). A number of researchers have recently emphasized that theory about human development has essentially been constructed on the basis of data only about men and then generalized to women. Women have often been considered "deviant" or a variant of the norm. Only recently has women's development been seen from the perspective of a different developmental path resulting in "primary" or positive femininity (Gilligan 1982; Stoller 1976). Women's experience was generally absent from theory building in psychology; for example, Horner (1972) found in the 1960s, when she did her research on fear of success, that data about women in a sample were usually discarded because they were so different and at variance with findings in men.

## Classic Psychoanalytic Theory

Freud (1905, 1925) postulated, on the basis of clinical experience with adults, that girls and boys developed similarly for the first few years until they became fully aware of the anatomical differences between them. He thought that children assumed that everyone started life with a penis and then, with the recognition of differences between boys and girls, discovered that the female body was "missing" a penis. This recognition constituted a "castration shock"; that is, the girl thought she had a penis originally and lost it, for which she blamed her mother, and was angry and envious and felt "castrated" or defective. The boy wondered if his angry, competitive, or early sexual feelings might result in punishment by castration, which would result in his becoming like a girl.

Freud saw this awareness of genital differences and their consequences as a turning point in the growth of the girl who moved away from her mother and toward her father. He viewed the girl's early development as essentially "masculine," with pleasurable sexual sensations deriving from her clitoris as parallel to the boy's phallic experiences. Her early relationship with her mother was profoundly affected by the discovery of this "inferiority." This disappointment also was believed to lead to a renunciation of masturbation and thus "active" sexuality for the little girl. Freud thought of the clitoris as an inferior, small penis, rather than a female organ of pleasure. He assumed that the girl experienced this in the same way and inevitably felt disappointed. He further hypothesized that the girl turned away from her mother (whom she devalued) when she realized that her mother did not have a penis either, and then turned toward her father, thus beginning the girl's oedipus complex. In the process, she gave up her earlier "activity," became more passive, and was left with lifetime penis envy.

Eventually, in the course of her development toward femininity, she gave up the wish for a penis and substituted the wish for a baby. Freud thought women inevitably wished for boy babies who would symbolically provide a penis. Thus the little girl, according to classical theory, was thought to have a devalued sense of her own body, which was to be compensated for by having a baby later.

For boys, the growing attachment to mother and rivalry with the father intensified the boy's anxiety and fear of punishment by castration. Castration anxiety was a powerful pressure for renouncing oedipal wishes for his mother and encouraging a more clear-cut and definite movement out of the oedipal phase, compared to the more fluctuating and less clear progression of this phase for the girl.

Superego development in boys was also thought to be different because of this process. Parental values were internalized in the process of moving out of the oedipal phase. The superego of the boy was more rigid and, Freud believed, "stronger." Freud's observations on women's "sense of justice" and morality included the belief that women had "little sense of justice because of the predominance of envy in their mental life" and that "they show less sense of justice than men. . . . They are less ready to submit to the great exigencies of life, they are more often influenced in their judgments by feelings of affection or hostility" (Freud 1925, pp. 257–258).

Women, he believed, had a difficult path toward maturation, and they were therefore not as creative nor did they contribute to civilization in the way that men did. He considered that women's responsiveness to the emotional demands of people close to them provided a potential for "corruption" of an abstract sense of fairness and justice. In addition, creative potential for women was fulfilled more directly by reproduction.

## Recent Psychoanalytic Views

These ideas have been challenged, and thinking has changed with more direct observation and data collection. The idea of the substitutive nature of the wish for a baby is no longer held, and it is now thought that a "core gender identity" exists (Money and Ehrhardt 1972; Stoller 1973), including the expectation of motherhood as part of a feminine self concept, although the adult woman may not become a mother. Although there are questions about the inevitable link between motherhood and femininity, for the young girl, the idea that her body can grow a baby is important (Notman and Lester 1988).

Current thinking has also challenged and changed some other concepts of development. For example, it has been questioned whether the girl turns away from the mother toward the father because she is disappointed in her mother. This action is probably more complexly determined by the girl's own growth and interest, her wish not to remain dependent, her father's interest in her, and maturation that de-idealizes both parents.

Current views of development hold that the establishment of a "gender identity" derives from many sources. Core gender identity, a newer concept, implies the perceptions of oneself as a girl or boy (Stoller 1968). Core gender identity begins to form with the initial parental recognition and labeling of the child as male or female. From the very beginning, parents and others relate differently to their infant daughters and sons. They speak to them differently, have different expectations, and present them with different communications and sets of signals and directions, which infants and children absorb and use as they build up mental representations of themselves. Children's anatomical and physical differences are important and interact with environmental experiences to build a male or female self concept.

The emergence of gender identity is observable by the time a child can speak, at about 18 months; it is considered to be irreversible at that time, and certainly by 3 years (Money and Ehrhardt 1972; Stoller 1968). Stoller (1976) discusses the stage of "primary femininity" that he believes precedes the oedipal period. This stage represents the little girl's conviction that she is "rightfully" female and feminine. Stoller holds that this is a conflict-free stage, the product of a firmly established core gender identity and a non-conflict-laden identification with feminine women. A later stage of development of femininity derives from the resolution of the oedipal period (Stoller 1976).

The toddler's understanding of self as being a girl or a boy, and what that means, is related to a number of experiences. The early relationships to the parents differ in boys and girls. For a girl, her identification with her mother is critical. She evolves a cognitive understanding of what "goes with" being a woman or a girl. For a boy to develop as masculine in our culture, he must abandon the affiliative and feminine style of the mother in favor of the more action-oriented, "instrumental," individualistic style of the male. The cognitive limitations of a child in this early stage of gender identity development do not permit the child to make a firm and entirely clear discrimination of one gender from another, that is, a total differentiation of girls and women from boys and men (Silverman 1981). However, the little girl recognizes that girls and women are grouped together because they "go together" on the basis of repeated communications and experiences. Also at this point, the idea that having babies is an activity of girls and women becomes established, particularly if the child has observed this. Boys must give up having babies as a direct possibility. In this way, both boys and girls give up something and eventually come to terms with their own potential.

The father is also important in this process. Fathers, no less than mothers, respond differently to female and male children. A little girl receives many cues from both parents, and her concept about being a girl is greatly influenced by what her father conveys to her about how he views her and about his feelings and attitudes about women. Similarly, cues and ideas of appropriate behavior for boys derive from parents and later from peers. It is in this context that genital awareness develops and the differences between girls and boys are recognized.

Direct observation indicates that there is distress when the child becomes aware of the anatomical difference between the sexes, and there is some degree of what has been interpreted as "narcissistic" injury for girls. However, how this distress is resolved will affect the importance of this problem in the adult woman. Galenson and Roiphe (1976) reported a definite response to the discovery of genital differences in young children observed as toddlers in a nursery school setting. They classified these responses as mild or intense castration reactions. Responses were mild when the child's earlier relationship to the mother was solid and earlier experiences were free of severe traumas and losses. If responses were severe, there generally was a "flawed" relationship to the mother or caregiver, or there had been some injury or loss of a parent or other important person or the recent birth of a sibling. The intense anxiety caused by these experiences leads to problems in development, such as heightening of an ambivalent tie to the mother, the absence of the shift to the father, and impoverishment of the girl's fantasy life. One can see the interplay of adequate early experiences of caregiving and nurturing with the degree of reaction to any sense of disappointment with one's body.

Lerner (1976) and Shopper (1979) point to the importance of parental mislabeling of the female genitals. The boy's genitals not only are easier to see but also are usually easier to label and it is easier to determine whether they are normal and like those of peers. A girl is usually told that she has a vagina, or a vagina and a uterus, which will bear babies later on. However, this is not what she is able to see when she looks down or in a mirror. She is not usually given labels for the vulva or for the clitoris, which is important in her pleasure. The fact that the girl's own exploration of her genitals is not corroborated or paralleled by information from her environment may lead to anxiety, confusion, and shame regarding her body and sexuality.

There has been much discussion of penis envy and its relationship to problems with self-esteem. The central theoretical position given to penis envy in classical psychoanalytical theory as a stimulus to feminine development has changed. It is no longer seen as occupying a pivotal position in adult women's psychological organization and development. It is considered a developmental experience rather than an inevitable and permanent feeling. If it is persistent it tends to be associated with other sources of envy in deprived women, such as losses and inadequate caregiving. The adult woman's feeling of defectiveness can be considered a fantasy organized around early childhood perceptions and a sense of narcissistic injury; manifestations of persistent penis envy in adult women can then be understood as failures of the developmental process (Grossman and Stewart 1976).

Early concepts of feminine development, for example, formulations by Helene Deutsch (1944), postulated a "normal" triad of feminine characteristics involving passivity, narcissism, and masochism. Masochism, as it was defined, was thought to represent an adaptation to the inevitable pain of childbirth and other feminine experiences. More recently, this hypothesis has been questioned and masochism has been viewed as unhealthy in either sex. Mature femininity is not seen as involving masochistic renunciation, but the capacity for love, nurturance, and sublimation (Blum 1976).

Although the complexities of individual and cultural differences in experience were recognized early by some authors as important determinants of concepts of femininity (Horney 1926; Thompson 1942, 1950; Zilboorg 1944), Freud (1925, 1931) did not accept these views for the most part; it has been left to more recent work to acknowledge these views. Recent criticism that the oedipal formulation in development is overemphasized has also focused attention on the importance of preoedipal ties and of the primary identification of the girl with her mother, an area that was relatively neglected earlier (Brunswick 1940; Chodorow 1978; Jones 1935; Klein 1945).

It has been proposed that because girls maintain their attachments to their mothers, a girl's gender identity is seen as continuous with her earliest identifications, whereas a boy's is not. It is the boy, then, whose developmental task can be seen as more complex and calling for object change and the need to reject feminine ties.

Passivity as a central aspect of adult femininity also does not include the normal, active maternal behavior with which the young child identifies and which has been recognized as "feminine" even in early psychoanalytic views. Conceptualizing femininity as identified with passive aims also does not include autonomous, assertive individuated development in women. Passivity, with changes in acceptable behavior for women in the past two decades, is perhaps less valid as a description of most women than it once was. Many women, however, do feel conflicted about being aggressive and do not easily use their abilities and talents. Conflicts about aggression persist clinically, although many women do not perceive them and others wish to change.

Narcissism was also part of the classical "feminine triad." Feminine narcissism was considered to be due to the girl's genital inferiority, in the early view. The term *narcissism* has acquired many new meanings. A normal degree of narcissism is considered important for adequate self-esteem for both men and women.

At any time in life, gender identity is inseparable from issues of self-esteem, although it is certainly not the only determinant. Individuals can feel good about themselves if they feel adequate as a man or woman, or as a girl or boy, no matter how these roles and functions are defined. Physical and sexual experiences, bodily gratifications, and acceptance of one's body and all its functions have been stressed as basic to the establishment of self-esteem.

### Adolescence

As development proceeds toward adolescence, children experience both interest and discomfort about the changes that take place in their bodies, accentuated by the unevenness of adolescent development (Petersen 1979). The degree of concern about the "rightness" of one's body can be intense, and fluctuations in self-esteem occur in response. Because girls and women have been seen as more oriented toward interpersonal relationships, they may be more sensitive to evaluations by peers and others. Boys are also concerned about how they measure up to others, which often takes the form of performance orientation and comparison. Gender identity and perception of gender roles in school-age children are strongly influenced by peers.

Menstruation is an important experience in girls' adolescent development. Kestenberg (1967) and others have observed that in early adolescence internal physical sensations and bodily changes are anxiety provoking. These feelings are unlocalized, and the inner sensations are undefined. Concern about one's normality can result. Earlier writers (Deutsch 1944) thought of the complex experience of menstruation as traumatic. Deutsch summarized much of the literature in her formulation that each period was a new disappointment at not being pregnant, revived ideas of genital injury, and reactivated old fears and conflicts about sexuality and masturbation. The mother's role toward her daughter contributed to these feelings, particularly the lack of preparation for menarche, which was the rule some time ago. Male attitudes toward menstruation have been primarily negative. Blood is associated with injury, and the menstrual blood can activate castration anxiety. Attitudes in many cultures reflect fear and danger associated with the menstrual cycle.

Kestenberg (1967) recognized the gamut of adult reaction to menstruation but questioned the inevitable traumatic aspect. She saw menarche as a potentially positive experience and as a turning point in the acceptance of femininity. Menstruation provided an "organizer and cornerstone of feminine identification" (Kestenberg 1967), which was better than the undefined inner sensations prior to it. There is clinical research and evidence of diminished anxiety with the onset of menarche, although there may be discomfort with the actual menstrual periods.

The relationship with the mother is important at the time of menarche. Menarche normally stimulates the girl's diminished dependency on the mother, identification with her as a reproductive prototype, and renewed interest in father and boys. In prepuberty the girl's interest in her body expresses itself in a variety of fantasies. Menarche provides the girl with fixed points of reference on which she can organize her experience. Menarche confirms the existence of the vagina and to some extent the uterus. At the same time, menarche is ambivalently regarded by many girls, especially if they are very young and do not entirely understand the process. Some girls also find the monthly periods a nuisance that interferes with their freedom (Whisnant and Zegnus 1975). Girls also look upon the menses as a valued sign of maturity, and it confirms the sense that they are functioning appropriately and becoming adults.

Boys experience similar body changes as they grow into adulthood. They begin to have erections and nocturnal emissions, which may produce confusion and guilt as well as pride and a sense of adulthood. However, there is no real equivalent to the "mysterious" aspect of menstruation with the potentially evocative and anxiety-producing response to the menstrual blood.

Breast development is also unique to girls, who grow an entirely different organ, the breast, in adolescence. The breasts are highly charged; symbolic of nurturance, fertility, adulthood, and sexuality; and important in body image and self-esteem. The girl's development thus includes two aspects of waiting for her mature body functioning—breast development and pregnancy, when the uterus becomes visible and functional. This "waiting" can be incorporated in the female ego.

A second separation-individuation phase in adolescence has been described (Blos 1979) in which old attachments to parents shift and new supports from peers and other identification models facilitate consolidation of identifications and the formation of an adult identity. The process involves considerable experimentation and forward movement combined with regression. New roles for both males and females are part of this process; that is, they have increased freedom to explore roles other than those rigidly defined by gender role stereotypes. Stereotypes remain hard to change in spite of increasing opportunities for women. The strength of unconscious identifications with parents accounts in part for this persistence. A girl who grows up with family and career choices can also feel confused because her mother, who is the model for how to be a woman, may have had narrower possibilities. This confusion can result in a sense of conflict about surpassing the mother. These conflicts sometimes emerge around career decisions and require further resolution. Other later concerns can include the balance between expectations in a couple, reproductive decisions, the actual interactions that take place with children and work, and the adaptations these situations require.

## References

Alpert J (ed): Psychoanalysis and Women. Hillsdale, NJ, Analytic Press, 1986

Bernay T, Cantor D (eds): The Psychology of Today's Woman. Hillsdale, NJ, Analytic Press, 1986

Blos P: The Adolescent Passage. New York International Universities Press, 1979

Blum H: Masochism, the ego ideal, and the psychology of women. J Am Psychoanal Assoc 24:157–191, 1976

Brunswick R: The pre-oedipal phase of the libido development. Psychoanal Q 9:293–319, 1940

Chodorow N: The Reproduction of Mothering: Psychoanalysis and the Sociology of Gender. Berkeley, University of California Press, 1978

Clower V: The acquisition of mature femininity. Paper presented at the Mahler Symposium, Philadelphia, PA, May 1987

Deutsch H: The Psychology of Women, Vol 1. New York, Grune & Stratton, 1944

Freud S: Three essays on the theory of sexuality (1905), in The Standard Edition of the Complete Psychological Works of Sigmund Freud, Vol 7. Translated and edited by Strachey J. London, Hogarth Press, 1953, pp 125–243

Freud S: Some psychical consequences of the anatomical distinction between the sexes (1925), in The Standard Edition of the Complete Psychological

Works of Sigmund Freud, Vol 19. Translated and edited by Strachey J. London, Hogarth Press, 1961, pp 248–260

Freud S: Female sexuality: introductory lectures on psychoanalysis (1931), in The Standard Edition of the Complete Psychological Works of Sigmund Freud, Vol 21. London, Hogarth Press, 1961, pp 223–243

Galenson E, Roiphe H: Some suggested revisions concerning early female development. J Am Psychoanal Assoc 24(5):29–57, 1976

Gilligan C: In a Different Voice. Cambridge, MA, Harvard University Press, 1982

Grossman W, Stewart W: Penis envy as metaphor. J Am Psychoanal Assoc 24:193–212, 1976

Horner M: Toward an understanding of achievement-related conflicts in women. Journal of Social Issues 28:157–173, 1972

Horney K: The flight from womanhood. Int J Psychoanal 7:324–339, 1926

Jones E: Early female sexuality. Int J Psychoanal 6:263–273, 1935

Kestenberg J: Phases of adolescence, parts I and II. J Am Acad Child Psychol 6:426–462, 1967

Klein M: The oedipus complex in the light of early anxieties (1945), in Love, Guilt, and Reparation and Other Works 1921–1945 (The Writers of Melanie Klein Ser). Edited by Money-Kyrle R. New York, Free Press, 1984, pp 370–419

Lerner H: Parental mislabelling of female genitals as a determinant of penis envy and learning inhibitions in women. J Am Psychoanal Assoc 24:269–284, 1976

Money J, Ehrhardt A: Man and Woman, Boy and Girl. Baltimore, MD, Johns Hopkins University Press, 1972

Notman M: Feminine development: changes in psychoanalytic theory, in The Woman Patient, Vol 2. Edited by Notman M, Nadelson C. New York, Plenum, 1982, pp 3–29

Notman M, Lester E: Pregnancy: Theoretical Considerations, Psychoanalytic Inquiry, Vol 8. Hillsdale, NJ, Analytic, 1988, pp 139–159

Petersen A: Female pubertal development, in Female Adolescent Development. Edited by Sugar M. New York, Brunner/Mazel, 1979, pp 23–46

Shopper M: The (re)discovery of the vagina and the importance of the menstrual tampon, in Female Adolescent Development. Edited by Sugar M. New York, Brunner/Mazel, 1979, pp 214–233

Silverman M: Cognitive development and female psychology. J Am Psychoanal Assoc 29:581–605, 1981

Stoller R: Sex and Gender. New York, Science House, 1968

Stoller R: Overview, the impact of new advances in sex research on psychoanalytic theory. Am J Psychiatry 132:241–251, 1973

Stoller R: Primary Femininity. J Am Psychoanal Assoc 24:59–78, 1976

Thompson C: Cultural pressures in the psychology of women. Psychiatry 5:331–339, 1942

Thompson C: Some effects of the derogatory attitude towards female sexuality. Psychiatry 13:349–354, 1950

Tyson P: A developmental line of gender identity, gender role, and choice of love object. J Am Psychoanal Assoc 30:61–86, 1982

Whisnant L, Zegnus L: A study of attitudes toward menarche in white middle class American adolescent girls. Am J Psychiatry 132:809–814, 1975

Zilboorg G: Masculine and feminine: some biological and cultural aspects. Psychiatry 7:257–296, 1944

# Chapter 10

# Epilogue

## Carol Gilligan, Ph.D.

It is a privilege to comment on the summaries of research from a wide range of disciplines, involving current findings on sex differences, and to reflect on assumptions and implications in light of data that researchers are gathering.[1]

In Chapter 1, Dr. LeVine says that anthropology always brings the counterexample to psychology. I certainly agree with him; I also think that anthropology brings a framework of tremendous value, particularly in dealing with the question of gender differences, in the sense that it calls attention to the fact that issues such as gender are constructed in a culture of meaning. One way to think about this discussion is to think about how psychiatry, psychology, and social science in general have become a culture within which gender has been constructed. Thus the question is not simply what are the gender differences and what can we learn by studying specific and often remote areas, but how can we become more reflective about the culture of studying gender within which all of us, in one way or another, practice and therefore perpetuate.

Anthropology offers a powerful analytic model in this discussion, especially since the social sciences have had a difficult time in dealing with the issue of gender. If one looks at the world in terms of the material presented here, one would think of gender as one variable among many; yet if one looks at psychological theory, gender seems to be the most problematic, the most difficult, or even a nonexistent variable. It is important, then, to become more reflective about our

Presented at the annual meeting of the American Psychiatric Association, Washington, DC, 1986.

own culture and our own methods and their implications for how we talk and think about gender, as well as how that itself shapes the role of gender during the life-cycle. When we develop quantitative scales, we leave ourselves little room to talk about differences except in terms of who is higher and who is lower. Thus there is an understandable tendency to shrink away from the kind of discussion that compares males and females and to hope that the whole issue of sex differences will go away.

Are there any surprises in this material? Do these studies present data not previously reported? Although there are clarifying refinements in certain areas, the terrain crossed is familiar. Because the areas where gender difference do and do not tend to show up are, in general, not surprising, the key question raised in this book is how to think about this latest evidence.

Dr. Russo, in Chapter 5, reminded us how much of our research has been "double blind," meaning blind to gender and blind to race. It is particularly difficult for psychologists to talk about sex differences because no one stands in a disinterested position.

Yet we must ask how research and therapy will differ if we attend to, rather than control for, sex and race. The questions not to ask have been delineated in this book. We are beyond asking the simplistic form of the question: Is it nature or is it nurture? Instead, we are beginning to frame more sophisticated questions about the interaction between biology, culture, and psychology. For example, hormones do not directly affect psychology or culture, but are mediated by psychology, culture, and therefore interpretation. The interpretive point was mentioned specifically with respect to the issue of labeling. One of the issues affecting the meaning of biological sex and psychological gender is how one speaks about them.

Some points are worthy of note. One is the continuing need to attend to the nonrepresentation of girls' and women's experiences in psychological research. We saw this need briefly in the studies of rhesus monkeys. Rough-and-tumble play—typically shown more by male monkey infants—could be increased by administering male sex hormones to female infants. But what about the female rhesus monkeys? What were they doing if they weren't doing rough-and-tumble play? It is important to ask what the females are doing and to watch closely the language one uses in representing female behavior.

Why are differences so difficult to talk about? In some sense if one thought about sex differences logically it would be odd to ask what kinds of psychological processes or psychological difficulty could be uninfluenced by sex or gender.

Although it seems difficult for psychologists to measure significant differences between women and men, this material suggests another approach. In Chapter 2, Dr. Kahne reports the continuing 60–70% disparity in income and earning power between men and women, which seems to have important implications for women's and men's psychology. How does this income disparity affect people? We might assume that such a disparity would have psychological ramifications; if we do not find it, what are the possible explanations?

Data on differences in verbal facility and in spatial ability do seem to appear frequently in the literature in this field. If we take such evidence seriously, we still must ask, "What does it mean? What are the psychological ramifications of girls having greater access, as a group, to verbal fluency and boys to spatial orientation?"

A few observations not addressed in this book are also pertinent. For example, Beatrice Whiting, an anthropologist, reports that most children, starting at about the age of 3 and increasing dramatically in the elementary school years, tend to play in same-sex peer groups (1988). Any differences between these groups—in their play or group structure—should have certain kinds of effects on children during middle childhood.

It appears to be easier to study biological factors than to study social, cultural, or psychological factors. Therefore, it is easier to amass biological evidence and then to create a picture that the data are essentially biological phenomena. This illustrates the culture of social science: what research is funded and what is supported create the reality that then influences the phenomenon.

It also seems to me that it is easier to study behavior and formulate theory that is typically associated with men, simply because males have been studied so much more. Therefore, there are more measures, a much larger vocabulary for describing male behavior, and more refined concepts or themes. As a result, it is easier to continue to elaborate those aspects of life that are traditionally male. In Chapter 7, Dr. Clower reminds us of this point, the psychoanalytic perspective. Likewise, to use Dr. Kahne's phrase, we speak of "paid work" in talking about the nature of work and work satisfaction. Looking at the areas of life traditionally associated with women, such as unpaid work, is more complex. Because these areas have not been studied, to even describe the phenomenon, one may have to start almost de novo and create the concepts, measurements, and vocabulary.

It also seems to me that we have to look at the consequences of the kinds of differences that have been cited. Can we formulate hypotheses about what might be the psychic consequences of earlier access to verbal or spatial skills and of the fact that women as a group tend to earn only 60–70% of male earnings? These observed psychological and sociological differences would seem to have implications for family interaction, marriage relationships, and divorce because they signify that men and women face different realities. Dr. Bernard develops this point in Chapter 8. If differences in earning power are not psychically represented, someone is out of touch with reality, which is a major psychological concern. In a sense, if one finds no psychological sex differences in these areas of documented economic sex differences, then you know what is not being psychically represented.

Finally, I will address current gaps and avenues for further research. One important area is the study of children and developmental sex differences, as Dr. Russo mentioned. Because children are being taken care of by the adult men and women living in the culture, it seems that we need to connect the study of sex differences on the level of child development and on the level of the experience of adult women and men. Finally, Dr. LeVine reminds us that the question will not go away, that if we ask, "Are there sex differences?" the answer is yes. If we ask, "Are there no sex differences?" the answer is yes and in a sense, to frame it simplistically, to ask, "Are there sex differences or not?" guarantees that we will get nowhere. He spoke of the obvious sex differences that we see in aggression and in who typically takes care of young children. These sex differences make everybody uncomfortable because they are easily translated to mean that all men should be aggressive and all women should stay home and take care of children.

This book is a giant step away from that kind of simplistic response. It is important not to get into trivial arguments about sex differences in specific skills when some major patterns of sex differences have clear psychic consequences that vary in different cultural settings and about which one cannot make simple statements or even foresee a simple way to understand. We now see recurrent patterns of sex differences, and therefore we have a greater opportunity to think about what they mean and to ask more intelligent questions. To think seriously about the implications of observations of sex differences and observations of no sex differences for education and therapy, it is also necessary to think about the place of sex and gender in the culture or the theoretical framework within which the activities of psychotherapy and education take place.

# Reference

Whiting B, with Edwards CP: Children of Different Worlds: The Formation of Social Behavior. Cambridge, MA, Harvard University Press, 1988

# Editors' Note

1. Current scholarship about gender differences and gender issues, within the tradition of feminist thinking, considers several important ideas. One idea involves the concept of gender as reflecting a series of culturally and socially shaped behaviors and norms. Although no one is so naive as to totally disregard biological differences, it sometimes appears that these differences are minimized and that the enormous influence of cultural patterns on the polarization that constitutes the concept of gender is emphasized. Dr. Gilligan addresses these concerns from a position that acknowledges and values gender differences. This position has also, at times, been considered "conservative," to reinforce old inequalities. Dr. Gilligan makes it clear, however, that this is not her position. Another trend in feminist scholarship has been to examine the degree to which social institutions reflect styles, norms, thinking, and values that are essentially masculine and thus represent the perspective of the dominant group in our society. The extent to which this is true is often not recognized by the clinician, and it is extremely important when one must assess the "normality" or pathology of a patient.

# Afterword

In the past decade there has been an increased awareness of the absence of data about gender differences in many fields. This awareness has stimulated investigation and led to greater understanding of the importance of considering gender in describing individual experiences. This body of data is still not widely recognized, and its incorporation into the literature is uneven and spotty. Our training facilities often do not include a curriculum in this area, or they teach it in a separate form, such as women's studies. Therefore, the integration of newer ideas and findings into general knowledge and theory has been delayed.

There are important clinical implications. For example, the ignorance of norms for women's experience results in inappropriate diagnostic categorization and treatment approaches. Sometimes the effect is more subtle, analogous to the lag in conceptualization that is the result of failure to integrate new knowledge into the thinking that pervades a field, such as the omission of findings about neurotransmitters from concepts of depression and anxiety.

Examples of the failure to integrate emerging knowledge are seen in the slow progress we make in shifting some of the traditional concepts of femininity and masculinity. For example, the role of work and family and concepts about the intuitive "rightness" of gender roles turn out, on closer inspection, to be specific to historical time and culture.

This volume is a sampling of the work that has been done in this area. We hope it will provide a wider knowledge as well as the basis for clinical application.

Malkah T. Notman, M.D.
Carol C. Nadelson, M.D.

# Index

Ability tests
  format, 48
  research problems, 47–48
Adaptation
  anthropology, 3
  gender-specific capacities, 3
  sexual dimorphism, 2–3
Adolescent development,
    123–125
  body changes, 124
  New Guinea, 6
  separation and individuation,
    125
Adultery, legal aspects, 108
Affirmative action legislation,
    14–15
Androgen-insensitivity
    syndrome, 26–27
Androgen secretion,
    development, 36
Anthropological data, 1–7
Anthropology, and psychology,
    129–130
Aptitude, biological genetic
    differences, 27
Auditory tests
  and hemispheric
    lateralization, 68
  research problems, 68–69
Awareness, infants, 32

Babies. *See* Infants

Behavior
  central nervous system
    organization, 28–29
  perinatal hormonal
    environment, 28–29
Bilateral representation, and
    age, 27
Biological and experiential
    basis of behavior,
    comparison, 26
Biological gender differences
  culture, 23
  hormones, 27
  neurological structure and
    function, 23–28
  research problems, 67
Bonding, in infants, 32
Brain
  cells, morphological
    differentiation and
    functional specialization, 39
  hemispheric lateralization, 24,
    25, 29–30, 66–67, 68,
    69–70
  hormones, 35–40
  sex hormones, 39–40
  structure, 23, 64

Caretaker expectations, 78
Castration anxiety, 81–82, 119
Cells, sex hormone effects,
    38–40